We would like to thank the following for their assistance in producing this edition of the Obstetric Guidelines on behalf of the Bedside Clinical Guidelines Partnership and Staffordshire, Shropshire & Black Country Newborn and Maternity Network

Contributors

Robina Akhtar
Krishna Banavathi
Jacqui Bolton
Junny Chan
Lynn Dudley
Jackie Dunn
Janet Herrod
Carol Hollington
Angela Hughes
Radha Indusekhar
Sarah Jamieson
Paddy McMaster
Rosamund Sawyer
Helen Sullivan

Obstetrics editors

Jacqui Bolton
Junny Chan
Helen Sullivan

Pharmacist

Helen Haley

Bedside Clinical Guidelines Partnership

Marian Kerr
Naveed Mustfa
Stephen Parton

Staffordshire, Shropshire & Black Country Newborn and Maternity Network

Sarah Carnwell
Ruth Moore

Patient representatives

Claire Anderson
Jennifer Barnes
Kate Branchett
Karen Cannon
Pippa Davies
Amanda Hartland
Mary Hayward
Brandi Jones
Sian Midwinter
Emma Raine
Karen Ramsey
Harriet Struthers
Becky Vintage

The editors would like to thank the following people/organisations for providing specialist information

Birmingham Women's Hospital – Fetal loss guideline

COMMONLY USED ABBREVIATIONS • 1/2

A

AAGBI	Association of Anaesthetists of Great Britain and Ireland
ABG	Arterial blood gas
ACEI	Angiotensin-converting enzyme inhibitor
AFE	Amniotic fluid embolism
AFP	Alpha-fetoprotein
ALS	Advanced life support
AN	Antenatal
ANC	Antenatal clinic
ANNP	Advanced neonatal nurse practitioner
APH	Antepartum haemorrhage
ARB	Angiotensin II receptor blockers
ARM	Artificial rupture of membranes

B

BBA	Born before arrival
BCG	Bacilli calmette-guerin
BD	Twice daily (BIS Die)
BLS	Basic life support
BMI	Body mass index
BO	Bowels opened
BP	Blood pressure
BPM	Beats per minute

C

CBD	Catheter bag drainage
Ceph	Cephalic
CESDI	Confidential enquiry into stillbirths and deaths in infancy
CMACE	Centre for maternal and child enquiries
CMACH	See CMACE
CMW	Community midwife
CPR	Cardio-pulmonary resuscitation
CRP	C reactive protein
CS	Caesarean section
CSU	Catheter specimen of urine
CVA	Cerebrovascular accident
CVP	Central venous pressure
CVS	Chorionic villus sampling
CX	Cervix
CXR	Chest X-ray

D

DIC	Disseminated intravascular coagulation
DNA	Did not attend
DFM	Diminished fetal movements
DS	Delivery suite
DVT	Deep venous thrombosis

E

EAS	External anal sphincter
EBL	Estimated blood loss
ECG	Electrocardiography
ECV	External cephalic version
EDD	Expected date of delivery
EFM	Electronic fetal monitoring
EGC	Emergency gynaecology clinic
ELLSCS	Elective lower segment caesarean section
EMLSCS	Emergency lower segment caesarean section
EPU	Early pregnancy unit
ERPC	Evaluation of retained products of conception

F

FBC	Full blood count
FBS	Fetal blood sampling
FHR	Fetal heart rate
FSE	Fetal scalp electrode

G

GBS	Group B *streptococcus*
GCS	Glasgow coma scale
G	Gravida
GTN	Glycerol trinitrate
GTT	Glucose tolerance test

H

Hb	Haemoglobin
HBIG	Hepatitis B immunoglobulin
HBV	Hepatitis B virus
Hcg	Human chorionic gonadotrophin
HCV	Hepatitis C virus
HDC	High dependency care
HDU	High dependency unit
HELLP	Haemolysis, elevated liver enzymes and low platelet count
H/O	History of
HVS	High vaginal swab

Issue 3
Issued: April 2015
Expires: April 2017

CONTENTS · 1/2

Guidelines

CONTENTS • 2/2

Issue 3
Issued: April 2015
Expires: April 2017

I

IAP	Intrapartum antibiotic prophylaxis
IAS	Internal anal sphincter
ICS	Intra-operative cell salvage
INR	International normalised ratio
IOL	Induction of labour
IPPV	Intermittent positive pressure ventilation
IUD	Intrauterine death
IUGR	Intrauterine growth restriction
IUT	Intrauterine transfer
IV	Intravenous
IVI	Intravenous infusion

L

LSCS	Lower segment caesarean section
LFT	Liver function tests
LGA	Large for gestational age
LMA	Laryngeal mask airway
LMP	Last menstrual period
LMWH	Low molecular weight heparin
LVS	Low vaginal swab

M

MAC	Minimum alveolar concentration
MAP	Mean arterial pressure
MAU	Maternal assessment unit
MBC	Midwife birth centre
MEOWS	See MEWS
MEWS	Maternity Early Warning Scoring
$MgSO_4$	Magnesium sulphate
MROP	Manual removal of placenta
MSSU	Midstream sample of urine

N

NAD	No abnormality detected
NEWS	Neonatal early warning score
NICE	National institute for clinical excellence
NICU	Neonatal intensive care unit
NIPE	Neonatal and infant physical examination
NLS	Neonatal life support

O

ODP	Operating department practitioner
OGTT	Oral glucose tolerance test

P

P	Parity
PCEA	Patient-controlled epidural anaesthesia
PE	Pulmonary embolism
PEA	Pulseless electrical activity
PET	Pre-eclamptic toxaemia
PIH	Pregnancy induced hypertension
PM	Post mortem
PN	Postnatal
PPH	Postpartum haemorrhage
PR	Per rectum
PROM	Pre-labour rupture of membranes
PV	Per vagina

Q

QDS	Four times daily

R

RCOG	Royal college of obstetricians and gynaecologists
RCM	Royal college of midwives
RCT	Randomised controlled trial
Rh	Rhesus
RM	Registered midwife

S

SGA	Small for gestational age
SROM	Spontaneous rupture of membranes
SVD	Spontaneous vaginal delivery

T

TEDS	Thromboembolic deterrent stockings
TOP	Termination of pregnancy

U

U&E	Urea and electrolytes
UKOSS	UK Obstetric Surveillance Survey
USS	Ultrasound scan
UTI	Urinary tract infection

V

VBAC	Vaginal birth after caesarean section
VE	Vaginal examination
VF	Ventricular fibrillation
VTE	Venous thromboembolism

This is the third edition of the Bedside clinical guidelines partnership/Staffordshire, Shropshire & Black Country Newborn and Maternity Network Obstetric guidelines. It has been compiled as an aide-memoire for all staff concerned with obstetric management, towards a more uniform standard of care.

The Staffordshire, Shropshire & Black Country Newborn and Maternity Network and the Bedside Clinical Guidelines Partnership have provided the logistical, financial and editorial expertise to produce these guidelines.

These guidelines have been drafted with reference to published medical literature and amended after extensive consultation. Wherever possible, the recommendations made are evidence based. Where no clear evidence has been identified from published literature the advice given represents a consensus of the expert authors and their peers and is based on their practical experience.

No guideline will apply to every patient, even where the diagnosis is clear-cut; there will always be exceptions. These guidelines are not intended as a substitute for logical thought and must be tempered by clinical judgement in the individual patient and advice from senior colleagues.

The guidelines are advisory, NOT mandatory

Supporting information

Where possible the guidelines are based on evidence from published literature. It is intended that evidence relating to statements made in the guidelines and its quality will be made explicit.

Where supporting evidence has been identified it is graded I to V according to standard criteria of validity and methodological quality as detailed in the table below. A summary of the evidence supporting each statement is available, with the original sources referenced. The evidence summaries are developed on a rolling programme which will be updated as the guideline is reviewed.

Level of evidence	Strength of evidence
I	Strong evidence from at least one systematic review of multiple well-designed randomised controlled trials
II	Strong evidence from at least one properly designed randomised controlled trial of appropriate size
III	Evidence from well-designed trials without randomisation, single group pre-post, cohort, time series or matched case-control studies
IV	Evidence from well-designed non-experimental studies from more than one centre or research group
V	Opinions of respected authorities, based on clinical evidence, descriptive studies or reports of expert committees

JA Muir-Gray from Evidence Based Healthcare, Churchill Livingstone London 1997

Evaluation of the evidence-base of these guidelines involves review of existing literature then periodical review of anything else that has been published since last review. The editors encourage you to challenge the evidence provided. If you know of evidence that contradicts, or additional evidence in support of, the advice given in these guidelines please forward it to the Clinical Guidelines Developer/Co-ordinator on bedsideclinicalguidelines@uhnm.nhs.uk

Feedback and new guidelines

The editors acknowledge the time and trouble taken by numerous colleagues in the drafting and amending of the text. The accuracy of the detailed advice given has been subject to exhaustive checks. However, any errors or omissions that become apparent should be drawn to the notice of the editors, via the Clinical Guidelines Developer/Co-ordinator bedsideclinicalguidelines@uhnm.nhs.uk, so that these can be amended in the next review, or, if necessary, be brought to the urgent attention of users. Constructive comments or suggestions would also be welcome.

The following guidelines are new to this edition:

- Extreme prematurity
- Morbidly adherent placenta
- Neurological deficits after regional anaesthesia or analgesia
- Stem cell banking
- Transcervical catheter induction

The following changes have been made:

- Clinical risk assessment guideline has been incorporated into the Labour management guideline

If there are any guidelines you would like to see in the next edition, please submit as soon as possible for editorial comment. The deadline for suggestions for revisions or new guidelines to be included will be November 2015

Effective communication is essential for delivery of high quality, safe care

COMMUNICATION

- Ensure information given to woman is presented in a way she can understand
- Maintain effective and appropriate communication with your colleagues

- Maintain knowledge and develop your abilities in team-based communication, keeping in mind the reliance placed on your communication and recording of information

DOCUMENTATION

- Record all discussions and actions relating to woman's care, including discussions where she has not been directly involved
- Ensure all entries in healthcare records are clear, accurate, legible and contemporaneous and attributed to a named person with an identifiable role
- Do not include:
- unnecessary abbreviations or jargon
- meaningless phrases
- irrelevant or offensive speculation
- irrelevant personal opinions regarding the woman

- Ensure any justifiable alteration to your own or other healthcare professional's documentation is clearly attributed to a named person with an identifiable role. Original entry and alteration must be clear, legible and auditable
- Healthcare record must include details of assessments, reviews, treatment and evidence of arrangements for future and continuing care, including information given to woman

Issue 3
Issued: April 2015
Expires: April 2017

GUIDELINES

These guidelines are advisory, NOT mandatory

INTRODUCTION

- In normal pregnancy, maternal plasma volume increases by up to 50%, red cell mass gradually increases by approximately 20% and haemoglobin (Hb) concentration drops. This normal physiological response may resemble iron deficiency anaemia
- Do not give routine iron and folic acid supplementation until anaemia diagnosed (using pregnant ranges)

DEFINITION

- Haemoglobin <110 g/L in the first trimester and <105 g/L in the second and third trimesters

> **Women who are known to be anaemic in labour must give birth in an obstetrician-led unit with appropriate precautions to reduce or manage blood loss**

RISK FACTORS

- Women with malabsorption syndrome, haemoglobinopathy, epilepsy requiring anticonvulsants and multiple pregnancies are at increased risk of folate deficiency
- offer iron and folic acid supplementation
- Other groups may have an increased risk based on dietary or cultural factors. Assess on an individual basis

Causes of anaemia in pregnancy

- Iron deficiency
- Folic acid deficiency
- Vitamin B$_{12}$ deficiency
- Haemoglobin variants
- Other causes
- exclude chronic illness [e.g. recurrent urinary tract infection (UTI), chronic inflammatory bowel disease]
- women born outside the UK or with a history of foreign travel
- consider less common causes (e.g. chronic infections and parasitic infections)

Symptoms and signs

- Pallor
- Lethargy
- Shortness of breath
- Weight loss
- Depression
- Nausea
- Vomiting
- Gingivitis
- Diarrhoea
- Raised pulse rate
- Thready pulse

DIAGNOSING IRON DEFICIENCY ANAEMIA

- Screen for anaemia at booking and 28 weeks' gestation unless otherwise indicated
- Screen for sickle cell and thalassaemia at booking
- Diagnose iron deficiency anaemia if mean corpuscular volume (MCV) <80 fl
- Check serum ferritin, serum iron and total iron binding capacity (TIBC) saturation. Iron deficiency indicated by:
- ferritin level of <15 micrograms/L
- serum iron level of <12 micromoles/L
- TIBC saturation of <15%

TREATMENT

Advice to women with anaemia

Life-style

- Avoid alcohol
- Stop smoking

Dietary advice

- Animal protein – well cooked red meat (avoid pre-cooked chilled meat, and liver)
- Eggs
- Milk
- Increase vitamin C to aid iron absorption (fresh orange juice, citrus fruits)

Issue 3
Issued: April 2015
Expires: April 2017

- Leafy green vegetables (not over-cooked)
- If concerns regarding compliance with dietary advice, give vitamin C as ascorbic acid 50 mg/day

TREATMENT OF IRON DEFICIENCY ANAEMIA

Aim of treatment

- Hb should rise by 20 g/L over 3–4 weeks

Elemental iron

- Give up to 100–200 mg elemental iron using one of the following preparations:
- ferrous sulphate 200 mg 8–12 hrly (ferrous sulphate contains 65 mg elemental iron per 200 mg tablet)
- ferrous fumerate 322 mg 12-hrly (each tablet contains 100 mg elemental iron)
- sodium feredetate 10 mL 8-hrly (contains 27.5 mg elemental iron per 5 mL dose)
- If these products are not tolerated, seek pharmacy advice

Side effects

- Advise woman that iron supplements may cause:
- gastrointestinal upset with nausea and epigastric pain
- where there is a history of constipation, use osmotic laxative

Monitoring

- Check haemoglobin 4 weeks after starting therapy
- an increase of 8 g/L/week is usual irrespective of the route of iron administration

Response to treatment

- Check compliance
- If not tolerant, try alternative preparations

- If inadequate response (<32 g/L)
- check iron studies, B12 and folate levels and refer to named consultant's antenatal clinic for next available appointment where IV iron therapy will be considered – see **Flowchart**
- In consultation with a haematologist, consider erythropoietin

Other forms of anaemia

- If MCV is >96 fl, consider other forms of anaemia

MACROCYTIC ANAEMIA

Definition

- Haemoglobin value and red cell numbers are reduced but MCV is increased
- In pregnancy, an MCV >96 fl is regarded as abnormal

Treatment

- Check levels of folate in blood and red blood cells and B_{12} levels in first instance
- If folate deficiency diagnosed, start folic acid 5 mg/day. Iron supplementation may also be necessary
- If B_{12} deficiency diagnosed, refer to GP or hospital antenatal clinic
- If both B_{12} and iron supplementation required, start B_{12} treatment first
- If folate and B_{12} levels are normal, refer to consultant antenatal clinic who will consider referral to haematology

Advice to woman

Lifestyle

- Avoid alcohol
- Stop smoking

Dietary

- Folic rich foods:
- leafy green vegetables (over boiling will destroy folic acid)
- chickpeas
- bananas
- citrus fruit
- avocado
- mushrooms
- asparagus
- bread and cereals fortified with folic acid

B_{12} deficiency known or diagnosed

- Eat animal protein – fresh well-cooked meat (avoid pre-cooked chilled meat)
- Well-cooked eggs
- Milk
- Cheese (avoid soft runny cheeses e.g., brie)
- Give vitamin B_{12} injections (hydroxocobalamin) 1 mg 3 times/week for 2 weeks, then 1 mg every 3 months according to response
- Take weekly red cell counts and haemoglobin estimations until a maintenance dose is reached
- Iron supplementation is prescribed as before in addition to vitamin B_{12} as rapid response to regeneration of red blood cells may deplete iron stores – see **Flowchart**

Anaemia flowchart

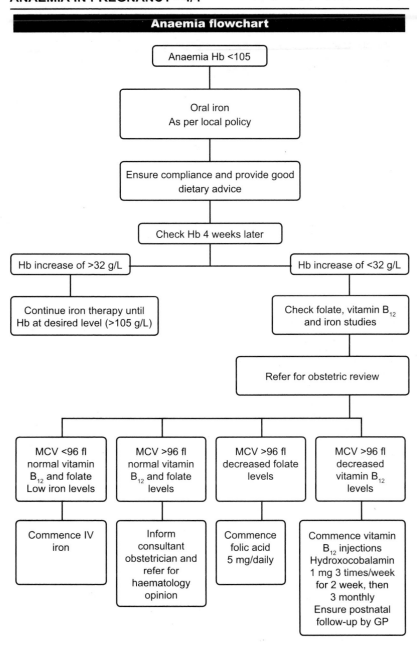

Anaemia Hb <105

↓

Oral iron
As per local policy

↓

Ensure compliance and provide good dietary advice

↓

Check Hb 4 weeks later

Hb increase of >32 g/L

Continue iron therapy until Hb at desired level (>105 g/L)

Hb increase of <32 g/L

Check folate, vitamin B_{12} and iron studies

↓

Refer for obstetric review

MCV <96 fl normal vitamin B_{12} and folate Low iron levels	MCV >96 fl normal vitamin B_{12} and folate levels	MCV >96 fl decreased folate levels	MCV >96 fl decreased vitamin B_{12} levels
Commence IV iron	Inform consultant obstetrician and refer for haematology opinion	Commence folic acid 5 mg/daily	Commence vitamin B_{12} injections Hydroxocobalamin 1 mg 3 times/week for 2 week, then 3 monthly Ensure postnatal follow-up by GP

ANTEPARTUM HAEMORRHAGE (APH)
(including placental abruption) • 1/3

DEFINITION

Bleeding from genital tract in woman of >24 weeks' gestation

INITIAL MANAGEMENT

- Admit to maternity unit
- Immediately assess severity of haemorrhage and whether immediate treatment required
- If maternal shock, marked abdominal pain or tenderness or fetal heart-rate abnormalities, see **Major APH or abruption** below
- Inform junior doctor and/or middle grade obstetrician (ST3–7 or equivalent e.g. staff grade, clinical fellow) who will review and formulate care plan
- Obtain detailed history from woman or those accompanying her
- Assess colour and amount of vaginal blood loss to determine whether fresh or stale, moderate or major bleed

Examination

- Full antenatal examination (in accordance with local Trust admission policy). Include:
- fundal height
- lie, presentation and 5ths palpable of presenting part. A high presenting part/abnormal lie can indicate placenta praevia
- examine abdomen for tenderness/tenseness/location of pain
- Perform vaginal speculum examination, except when known major placenta praevia
- Assess cervix dilatation and appearance
- Take triple swabs, including chlamydia
- Refer to ultrasound scan to determine location of placenta

> *If placenta low lying, do NOT perform digital vaginal examination to avoid accidental trauma to placenta and possible severe haemorrhage*

- Auscultate fetal heartbeat to determine presence

- Perform electronic fetal monitoring (EFM) to assess fetal wellbeing – see **Electronic fetal monitoring** guideline

> *If minor APH progresses to major, caesarean section indicated*

Monitor

- Start Maternity Early Warning Scoring chart (MEWS) – follow local procedure

Investigation

- Take bloods for:
- FBC
- group and save and crossmatch if significant bleed
- consider coagulation studies
- in Rhesus negative women, perform Kleihauer test to quantify the degree of any fetomaternal haemorrhage and determine dose of anti D required. It is of little value in diagnosing abruption

> *For Rh negative women, obstetrician will prescribe anti-D immunoglobulin*

MAJOR APH OR ABRUPTION

Presenting symptoms

- Maternal shock
- Marked abdominal pain or tenderness
- Fetal heart-rate abnormalities
- Bleeding may be concealed or revealed

MANAGEMENT

> *This is an obstetric emergency*

- Activate emergency buzzer and request assistance from:
- delivery suite team leader
- middle grade obstetrician (ST3–7 or equivalent e.g. staff grade, clinical fellow) and SHO
- on-call obstetric anaesthetist and anaesthetic nurse or operating department practitioner
- Notify consultant obstetrician and consultant anaesthetist
- Team leader will delegate management tasks and nominate a team member to document events

Issue 3
Issued: April 2015
Expires: April 2017

Resuscitation

- Manage and maintain – Airway, Breathing, Circulation
- Record vital signs every 5 min (include MEWS)
- Avoid aortocaval compression
- Give high flow oxygen

Replace blood volume loss

- Insert 2 large bore (14 or 16 gauge) IV cannulae
- Take blood for:
  - crossmatch
  - FBC
  - clotting screen
- Request blood and blood products urgently according to Trust Major haemorrhage protocol
- While awaiting blood, infuse compound sodium lactate (Hartmann's) solution or sodium chloride 0.9% and colloid
- If blood loss life-threatening un-crossmatched O Rhesus-negative blood or group-specific blood (if available) may be used from delivery suite blood refrigerator
- Insert indwelling urinary catheter

> ***When infusing large amounts of intravenous fluids rapidly, infuse via blood warmer***

Analgesia

- Dosage and administration according to severity of pain. Opiates may be required for placental abruption

Monitor

- BP
- Respiratory rate
- Pulse oximetry
- Renal function: monitor urine output hourly
  - report volume <30 mL/hr to attending obstetric and anaesthetic staff
- Fetal heart by EFM
  - if no signs of fetal heart-rate – ultrasound scan to confirm/rule out intrauterine death

Intrauterine death

- Inform consultant obstetrician and discuss plan of care with woman, considering severity of haemorrhage and maternal condition
- The longer the fetus stays in-utero, the higher the risk of disseminated intravascular coagulation (DIC)

Caesarean section

- If fetal heart-rate present and maternal condition stable, transfer to theatre for emergency caesarean section
- Inform neonatologist and request attendance at delivery

> ***Expect and be prepared for massive postpartum haemorrhage (PPH) whether delivered vaginally or by lower segment caesarean section (LSCS) – see* Postpartum haemorrhage *guideline***

- Central venous pressure (CVP) line/arterial line may be inserted by anaesthetic team to monitor fluid balance and aid resuscitation
- In coagulopathy or massive transfusion, seek advice from consultant haematologist, who will arrange blood and blood products and correct clotting factor deficiencies

Post-operative/ Post-delivery care

- Transfer woman to delivery suite high dependency area
- If ventilation necessary, transfer to acute Trust ITU – see **Maternal transfer** guideline

PLACENTA PRAEVIA

Definition

- Placenta wholly or partially inserted in lower segment of uterus

Major or complete

- Placenta encroaching on cervical opening (determined by ultrasound scan)
  - deliver by caesarean section

Minor or partial

- Placenta not encroaching on cervical opening

Management of bleeding

- Woman to remain on delivery suite
- Crossmatch minimum of 2 units of blood to delivery suite blood bank urgently

Conservative management

- Administer corticosteroids (in accordance with local policy) to assist fetal lung maturity
- In a significant bleed, on-call consultant obstetrician will discuss plan of care for conservative management or delivery with mother and document in maternal healthcare record

Caesarean section

- With significant bleeding, consultant obstetrician will deliver by caesarean section or directly supervise a middle grade obstetrician (ST3–7 or equivalent e.g. staff grade, clinical fellow), if available locally, consider cell salvage
- Crossmatch 4 units of blood and have ready in delivery suite blood bank, preferably before delivery achieved or, if available, group-specific blood

> *Women with a previous caesarean section and anterior placenta praevia are at high risk of placenta accreta and should be managed by consultant obstetrician and anaesthetist*

Choice of anaesthesia

- Decided by anaesthetist and woman – usually spinal but, in haemodynamically unstable woman, general anaesthesia may be indicated

Post-operative infusion

- Commence oxytocin infusion as per local practice

PLACENTA ABRUPTION

Definition

- Accidental haemorrhage due to partial or complete separation of normally situated placenta
- Bleeding may be concealed or visible

Risk factors

- Trauma
- Hypertensive disease or pre-eclampsia
- Previous abruption
- High parity
- Twin gestation
- Polyhydramnios
- Smoking
- Prolonged rupture of membranes

Management

Dependent on severity of bleed

- If minor APH, midwife will monitor:
- amount of vaginal blood loss
- abdominal tenderness
- pain
- vital signs
- If active bleeding, monitor fetus with continuous EFM

Conservative management

- Administer corticosteroids (in accordance with local policy) to assist fetal lung maturity
- If bleeding continues, consultant obstetrician/middle grade obstetrician (ST3–7 or equivalent e.g. staff grade, clinical fellow) will consider delivery, possibly by induction

EXTRAPLACENTAL BLEEDING

- Coagulation defects (e.g. von Willebrand's disease), cervical polyps, cervical ectropion, cervical infection, cervical carcinoma, ruptured vulval varices and infection

Issue 3
Issued: April 2015
Expires: April 2017

BACKGROUND

- Childbirth has the potential to cause long-term damage to the pelvic floor, affecting bladder or bowel function

- Most women have the urge to void within 6 hr postpartum

- 10–15% of women experience voiding dysfunction to some degree and for some time following delivery

- 5% have significant and longer lasting dysfunction

- this may lead to bladder over-distension and overflow incontinence with long-term significant bladder dysfunction

BLADDER DYSFUNCTION

Women at highest risk

- Primigravida

- Prolonged labour, especially prolonged second stage

- Epidural for labour and delivery

- Frequent catheterisation during labour

- Assisted vaginal delivery

- Caesarean section

- Perineal injury

- Big baby >4.5 kg

- Previous bladder problems (required individualised management plan for labour and puerperium)

Symptoms and signs

- Frequency/urgency/lower abdominal pain

- Prolonged voiding

- No sensation to void or inability to void

- Palpable bladder

- Overflow incontinence

ANTENATAL CARE

First antenatal visit

- Ask woman if she has ever experienced problems with bowel or bladder function. This can result in early detection of bladder/bowel dysfunction

- document response in medical history section of maternal healthcare record

- if problem highlighted, refer to appropriate healthcare professional (e.g. physiotherapist, urotherapist or consultant obstetrician) for plan of action

- Discuss:

- pelvic floor and urethral sphincter exercise

- diet to prevent constipation

Third trimester antenatal visit

- It is good practice to ask again if woman has ever experienced problems with bowel or bladder function. Women are often reluctant to disclose symptoms

MANAGEMENT IN LABOUR

First stage

- Encourage 2–4 hrly voiding

- threshold for catheterisation (in/out) should be low if woman unable to void on two occasions (after 4 hr) or maternal bladder is palpable

- if any void measures >500 mL, bladder should be emptied more frequently to prevent over-distention

- Maintain adequate hydration during labour

- Urinalysis with dipstick every void and document in partogram

Second stage

A full bladder may hinder descent of presenting part

- Ensure bladder is empty. If necessary, catheterise
- Bladder must be empty before instrumental delivery

POSTPARTUM CARE

Most women will experience supra pubic discomfort as their bladder distends but lack of this sensation does not mean the bladder is not full

- Encourage woman to void before leaving delivery suite
- Palpate abdomen for signs of palpable bladder, or deviation of uterus which may indicate urinary retention
- Record time and volume of first void in maternal healthcare record
- if volume >150–200 mL and woman experiences no difficulty in micturation or any other urinary symptoms, cease recording
- if volume <150 mL, see **Voiding small amounts of urine** below
- If clinical suspicion of dehydration, encourage fluids
- If no dehydration and retention suspected, do not encourage fluids as this can exacerbate retention. Seek advice from junior doctor and/or middle grade obstetrician (ST3–7 or equivalent e.g. staff grade, clinical fellow)
- establish when woman last passed urine in labour

Voiding small amounts of urine

- If woman continues to void small volumes of urine (<150 mL) 6 hr post-delivery, insert size 12 Foley catheter
- Measure residual urine volume or use bladder volume ultrasound screening if available

- if 200 mL, leave catheter in place freely draining for 24 hr and start a fluid balance chart
- if <150 mL, encourage increased fluid intake
- record amount of urine passed
- inform middle grade obstetrician (ST3–7 or equivalent e.g. staff grade, clinical fellow)
- Remove catheter after 24 hr and, if infection suspected, send catheter specimen of urine (CSU) for analysis
- rapid diuresis may occur and will depend on how much fluid has been consumed or infused
- measure next two voids. If >150 mL, discharge woman
- Repeat question – has woman ever experienced problems with bowel or bladder function
- document response in appropriate section of maternal healthcare record and management plan

Failure to void

- If unable to void 6 hr post-delivery, insert size 12 Foley urethral catheter
- Allow catheter to drain for 20 min then measure residual urine drained and document in maternal healthcare record and fluid balance chart or, if available, use bladder volume scanning
- Leave catheter in place for 24 hr
- Inform middle grade obstetrician (ST3–7 or equivalent e.g. staff grade, clinical fellow)
- Remove catheter after 24 hr and, if infection suspected, send CSU for analysis

If catheterisation required, women on midwife-led unit must be transferred to consultant-led unit

Continuing small volumes

- If still unable to void or continuing to void small volumes after catheter removal, inform consultant obstetrician

- Measure residual urine volume or, if available, use bladder volume screening

- if <150 mL, consider repeating residual volume measurement in 12 hr

- if >300 mL, replace indwelling catheter for at least 48 hr and, more commonly, 7 days

- if between 150–300 mL, discuss with woman and agree course of action, depending on her individual circumstances (e.g. repeat residual volume measurement after next void or insert catheter)

- Discuss management plan with woman and document in maternal healthcare record

- Arrange follow-up at six weeks postpartum e.g. in pelvic floor clinic

POSTNATAL CARE

- Ask again if woman has ever experienced problems with bowel or bladder function. Document response in appropriate section of maternal healthcare record. If problem highlighted, document in management plan and refer to appropriate healthcare professional (e.g. physiotherapy, urotherapist)

- Provide advice on:

- diet and fluids

- importance of avoiding constipation

- pelvic floor exercises

- simple analgesia

INTRODUCTION

In appropriate cases, caesarean section can be life-saving or can prevent serious morbidity to mother and fetus

CLASSIFICATION AND TIMING OF CAESAREAN SECTION

- Use classification below to communicate degree of urgency to all staff and ensure caesarean section is undertaken within an acceptable timeframe
- Prepare for a caesarean section to minimise risks of procedure and optimise mother's and her birth partner's experience. The shorter the decision to delivery interval the less optimal the preparation

Category	Definition	Standard
1 – Crash	Immediate threat to life of woman and fetus	Interval between decision to delivery time should not exceed 30 min
2 – Urgent	Maternal or fetal compromise not immediately life-threatening	Interval between decision to delivery time according to local practice
3 – Scheduled	Early delivery necessary – no maternal or fetal compromise	Interval between decision to delivery time according to local practice
4 – Elective	No maternal or fetal compromise	Undertaken at a time to suit both woman and obstetric team

CATEGORY 1 CAESAREAN SECTION

Preparation

- Middle grade obstetrician (ST3–7 or equivalent e.g. staff grade, clinical fellow) decides if caesarean section indicated and confirms with consultant as soon as possible
- Follow local practice to summon theatre team and inform category 1 caesarean section
- Transfer to theatre immediately
- Provide woman with as much information as possible and obtain consent
- verbal consent is acceptable in cases of extreme emergency
- Ensure blood taken for the following and deliver to laboratory urgently:
- full blood count (FBC)
- group and save

Documentation

- Person making decision for caesarean section documents the following in intrapartum care record
- indication and classification of emergency caesarean section
- time decision for caesarean section made
- reason for any delay in performing caesarean section
- Complete the WHO 'Five steps to safer surgery' theatre check list

Midwife

- Remove woman's jewellery or cover under adhesive tape
- Remove woman's nail polish
- If oxytocin infusion is running, switch off
- Attach patient identification (e.g. band) according to local practice

Issue 3
Issued: April 2015
Expires: April 2017

Anaesthetist

- Pre-assesses woman (may be continued en-route to and/or in theatre)
- Establish IV access 16 G cannula (if not already done)
- Give antacid treatment as per local policy

Theatre team

- Prepares theatre

In theatre

Anaesthetist, theatre team and midwife

- Place woman in left lateral tilt on operating table; commence oxygen
- Maternal monitoring – BP, ECG, oximetry
- Regional or general anaesthesia administered
- Administer prophylactic antibiotics as per local guidance
- Catheterise woman
- Check resuscitaire and emergency neonatal resuscitation equipment
- Call neonatal team to attend
- Obtain paired cord gases – see **Umbilical cord sampling** guideline or follow local practice

CATEGORY 2, 3 AND 4 CAESAREAN SECTION

Preparation

- There is more time for preparation e.g:
- more detailed explanation to woman and written consent
- dressing woman in hospital gown, hat to cover long hair
- fetal heart monitoring
- administer antacids as per local policy
- WHO 'Five steps to safer surgery' checklist

Obstetrician

- Provides detailed information to woman and obtains written consent
- Documents indication for emergency caesarean section in intrapartum maternal healthcare record
- Prescribes antacids as per local policy
- Commences caesarean section audit form (if local practice)

Anaesthetist

- Pre-assesses woman

Midwife

- Review woman's birth plan
- If not already arranged, ensure a midwife is allocated to care for the woman
- Midwife ensures:
- continuous electronic fetal monitoring (category 2) until surgery begins
- pre-operative check list completed
- VTE thromboprophylaxis as per local policy
- patient identification completed and *in situ*
- blood for FBC and group and save

FOLLOWING CAESAREAN SECTION

Obstetrician

- Completes caesarean section audit form (if local practice)
- Documents procedure in intrapartum maternal healthcare record according to local Trust procedure

Anaesthetist

- Transfers woman to recovery room
- Ensures appropriate antibiotic prophylaxis/analgesia/thromboprophylaxis prescribed
- Hands over to midwife/recovery nurse

Midwife/recovery nurse

- Recovery observations as per local practice

- Initiates skin-to-skin contact

- Completes appropriate documentation

IMMEDIATE/24 HOUR POST-OPERATIVE CARE

- Refer to local guidelines:

- post anaesthetic care within the maternity unit

- postnatal care within the maternity unit

Communication

- Obstetrician should discuss procedure with woman, offering advice about vaginal birth after caesarean section (VBAC). If local practice, give VBAC information leaflet

Documentation

- Obstetric medical staff to document need for follow-up in maternal healthcare record

- Check equipment daily, and before resuscitation
- Follow Resuscitation Council UK Guidelines www.resus.org.uk

DRY AND COVER

- Cord clamping – see **Cord clamping** below
- ≥28 weeks' gestation, dry baby, **remove wet towels** and cover baby with **dry towels**
- <28 weeks' gestation, do not dry body but place baby in plastic bag feet first, dry head only and put on hat

Cord clamping

- If baby does not require immediate resuscitation, clamp cord after 1 min
- If immediate resuscitation is required following assessment, clamp cord as soon as possible

ASSESS

- Assess **colour, tone, breathing and heart rate**

> *If baby very floppy and heart rate slow, assist breathing immediately*

- Reassess every 30 sec throughout resuscitation process
- If help required, request immediately

> *If baby not breathing adequately by 90 sec, assist breathing*

CHECK AIRWAY

> *For baby to breathe effectively, airway must be open*

- To open airway, place baby supine with head in **'neutral position'**
- If very floppy, give chin support or jaw thrust while maintaining the neutral position

IMMEDIATE TREATMENT

Airway

- Keep head in neutral position
- Use T-piece and soft round face mask, extending from nasal bridge to chin
- Give 5 inflation breaths, sustaining inflation pressure (**Table 1**) for 2–3 sec for each breath
- Give PEEP of 5 cm H_2O
- Begin inflation breaths in air

Table 1: Inflation pressure (avoid using pressure higher than recommended)

Term baby	30 cm of water
Preterm baby	20–25 cm of water

No chest movement

Ask yourself:

- Is head in neutral position?
- Is a jaw thrust required?
- Do you need a second person to help with airway to perform a jaw thrust?
- Is there an obstruction and do you need to look with a laryngoscope and suck with a large-bore device?
- Consider placing oro-pharyngeal (Guedel) airway under direct vision using laryngoscope
- Is inflation time long enough?
- if no chest movement occurs after alternative airway procedures **above** have been tried (volume given is a function of time and pressure), a larger volume can be delivered if necessary by inflating for a longer time (3–4 sec)
- Attach saturation monitor to right hand – see **Saturation monitoring** for guidance on SpO_2 targets

Endotracheal intubation

Indications

- Severe hypoxia (e.g. terminal apnoea or fresh stillbirth)
- Stabilisation of airway
- Extreme prematurity
- Congenital diaphragmatic hernia

Safe insertion of endotracheal tube requires skill and experience
If you cannot insert a tracheal tube within 30 sec, revert to mask ventilation
Capnography can help to assess endotracheal tube placement

Breathing

- Most babies have a good heart rate after birth and establish breathing by 90 sec
- if not breathing adequately give **5 inflation breaths**, preferably using air at pressures in **Table 1**
- Heart rate should rapidly increase as oxygenated blood reaches heart

Do not move onto ventilation breaths unless you have a heart rate response OR you have seen chest movement

Review assessment after inflation breaths

- Is there a rise in heart rate?
- Is there chest movement with the breaths you are giving?
- If no spontaneous breathing, but chest movement has been obtained, perform 30 sec of **ventilation breaths**, given at a rate of 30 breaths/min (1 sec inspiration)

Table 2: Outcome after 30 sec of ventilation breaths

Heart rate	Breathing	Action
Increases	Not started breathing	• Provide 30–40 breaths/min • Where available, use PEEP at 5 cm water with T-piece system
<60	Obvious chest movement	• Start chest compressions (see below)

- If baby is floppy with slow heart rate and there is chest movement, start cardiac compressions with ventilation breaths immediately after inflation breaths
- Increase inspired oxygen concentration every 30 sec by 30% e.g. 30–60–90% depending on response – see **Saturation chart**

Issue 3
Issued: April 2015
Expires: April 2017

Chest compression

● Use if heart rate approximately <60 beats/min (do not try to count accurately as this will waste time)

> *Start chest compression only after successful inflation of lungs*

Figure 1

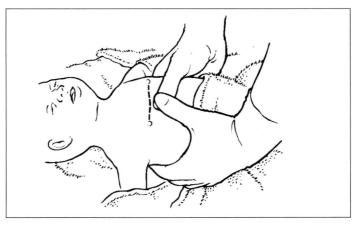

Figure 2

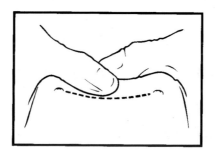

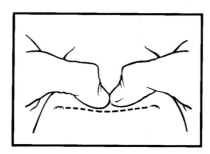

Pictures taken from NLS manual and Resuscitation Council (UK) and reproduced with their permission

Ideal hold (figure1/figure 2)

- Circle chest with both hands so that thumbs can press on the sternum just below an imaginary line joining the nipples with fingers over baby's spine

Alternative hold (less effective)

- Compress lower sternum with fingers while supporting baby's back. The alternative hand position for cardiac compressions can be used when access to the umbilicus for UVC catheterisation is required, as hands around the chest may be awkward

Action

- Compress chest quickly and firmly to reduce the antero-posterior diameter of the chest by about one-third, followed by full re-expansion to allow ventricles to refill

- remember to relax grip during IPPV, and feel for chest movement during ventilation breaths, as it is easy to lose neutral position when cardiac compressions are started

> *Co-ordinate compression and ventilation to avoid competition. Aim for 3:1 ratio of compressions to ventilations and 90 compressions and 30 breaths (120 'events') per min*

Blood

- If there is evidence of fetal haemorrhage, consider giving O negative emergency blood

Resuscitation drugs

- Always ask about drugs taken recently by, or given to mother

- Give drugs only if there is an undetectable or slow heartbeat despite effective lung inflation and effective chest compression

- Umbilical venous catheter (UVC) is the preferred route for urgent venous access

- Recommence cardiac compressions and ventilation breaths ratio 3:1 after each drug administration and re-assess after 30 sec

- If no heart rate increase, progress to next drug

Adrenaline 1:10,000

- 10 microgram/kg (0.1 mL/kg) IV

- If this dose is not effective, give 30 microgram/kg (0.3 mL/kg) after sodium bicarbonate has been given

- Adrenaline should only be given via the ET tube (ETT) if venous access is taking time to achieve; it should not delay intravenous access and treatment; the dose is 0.5–1.0 mL/kg of 1 in 10,000

Sodium bicarbonate 4.2%

- 1–2 mmol/kg (2–4 mL/kg) IV (never give via ET tube)

Glucose 10%

- 2.5 mL/kg IV slowly over 5 min

Sodium chloride 0.9%

- 10 mL/kg IV

Naloxone

- Give only after ventilation by mask or ETT has been established with chest movement seen and heart beat >100 beats/min

- If mother has been given pethidine within 2–4 hr of delivery, give IM naloxone:

- 100 microgram (0.25 mL) for small preterm babies

- 200 microgram (0.5 mL) for all other babies

WHEN TO STOP

- If no sign of life after 10 min, outlook is poor with few survivors, majority will have cerebral palsy and learning difficulties

- If no sustained spontaneous breathing 30 min after a heart rate has been established, majority also have poor prognosis

Continue resuscitation until a senior neonatologist advises stopping

MONITORING

Saturation monitoring

- Oxygen monitoring is activated when neonatologist/2nd pair of hands arrives. In the meantime, the person initiating resuscitation carries out all the usual steps in resuscitation

- Do not stop resuscitation for a saturation probe to be attached

- Attach saturation probe to the right hand and connect to the monitor once 5 inflation breaths have been given

- SpO_2 should spontaneously improve as **Table 3**

Table 3

Time (min)	Acceptable pre-ductal SpO_2 (%)
2	60
3	70
4	80
5	85
10	90

Air to oxygen

- If inflation breaths produce a response and SpO_2 monitoring is available with a reliable trace target, saturations as in **Table 3**

- If inflation breaths have been successful and chest movement seen but colour/SpO_2 (if available) not improved, increase oxygen to 30%

- If no response, increase by increments of 30% every 30 sec i.e:

  Term air: 30–60–90/100%

  Preterm air: 30– 60–90%

- If chest compressions are required following chest movement with inflation breaths, increase oxygen to 90%

- If SpO_2 above levels in **Table 3** or >95% at 10 min of life, reduce oxygen

Preterm deliveries

- ≥26 weeks' gestation do not require routine intubation if respiratory effort good

- these babies can receive PEEP at 5 cm H_2O via mask ventilation with oxygen supplementation as appropriate on the resuscitaire continuing PEEP support on transfer to NICU

- If respiratory effort is poor, at any point, or baby's condition deteriorates, intubate and ventilate

DOCUMENTATION

- Make accurate written record of facts (not opinions) as soon as possible after the event

- **Record**

- when you were called, by whom and why

- condition of baby on arrival

- what you did and when you did it

- timing and detail of any response by baby

- date and time of writing your entry

- a legible signature

COMMUNICATION

- Inform parents what has happened (the facts)

Newborn life support algorithm

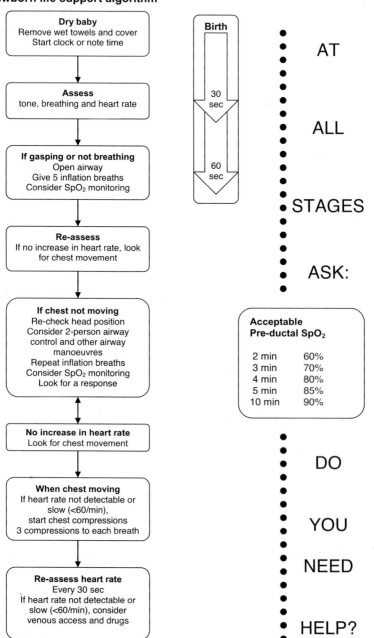

Dry baby
Remove wet towels and cover
Start clock or note time

↓

Assess
tone, breathing and heart rate

↓

If gasping or not breathing
Open airway
Give 5 inflation breaths
Consider SpO_2 monitoring

↓

Re-assess
If no increase in heart rate, look
for chest movement

↓

If chest not moving
Re-check head position
Consider 2-person airway
control and other airway
manoeuvres
Repeat inflation breaths
Consider SpO_2 monitoring
Look for a response

↓

No increase in heart rate
Look for chest movement

↓

When chest moving
If heart rate not detectable or
slow (<60/min),
start chest compressions
3 compressions to each breath

↓

Re-assess heart rate
Every 30 sec
If heart rate not detectable or
slow (<60/min), consider
venous access and drugs

Birth

30 sec

60 sec

AT

ALL

STAGES

ASK:

**Acceptable
Pre-ductal SpO_2**

2 min	60%
3 min	70%
4 min	80%
5 min	85%
10 min	90%

DO

YOU

NEED

HELP?

Issue 3
Issued: April 2015
Expires: April 2017

INTRAPARTUM PREPARATION

- Identify risk factors that may affect immediate care and devise management plan
- Ensure delivery room warm
- Check resuscitation equipment
- Pre-warm towels
- Summon multidisciplinary team members necessary for delivery and inform of risk factors

IMMEDIATE CARE

At delivery

- If baby does not require immediate resuscitation, clamp cord after 1 min
- If immediate resuscitation is required following assessment, clamp cord as soon as possible
- Dry with warm towel and cover to prevent heat loss
- Assess wellbeing and, if necessary, resuscitate – see **Cardiopulmonary resuscitation of the newborn** guideline
- Assess Apgar score at 1 and 5 min as a minimum. Document in intrapartum record
- If Apgar score at birth ≤5, continue to assess and record every 5 min. Document any appropriate action taken until score is ≥6 or baby is transferred to neonatal care
- If baby delivered in poor condition or risk factors identified during intrapartum period:
- double clamp cord and take cord blood for paired cord samples – see **Umbilical cord sampling** guideline
- inform neonatal team of abnormal results e.g. pH level <7
- Encourage first breast feed within 1 hour and skin-to-skin contact for at least 1 hour

- Avoid performing routine postnatal procedures during first hour after birth unless requested by mother or treatment necessary for wellbeing of baby
- Identify babies at increased risk of hypothermia (<37 weeks or small for dates) and hypoglycaemia (<37 weeks or <2.5 kg, babies of diabetic mothers)

Registration and identification

- Register and identify baby and mother as soon as possible. See **Registration and identification** section

THERMOREGULATION AND MANAGEMENT

> *Baby's temperature in normal room environment should be 37ºC*

- Encourage uninterrupted skin-to-skin contact with mother (or partner if appropriate)
- document offer and whether accepted by mother in intrapartum record. If declined or not done, note reasons
- Check baby's initial axillary temperature using digital thermometer while cradled by mother/partner (ideally 1–2 hr following birth). Record in intrapartum record
- If temperature ≥36.4°C, do not recheck axilla temperature unless:
- specific risk factors e.g. small for dates, preterm, maternal pyrexia during labour, group B *streptococcus* (GBS), pre-labour spontaneous rupture of membranes (PROM) – see **Group B streptococcus** guideline and **Pre-labour rupture of membranes (PROM)** guideline
- baby unwell
- Use digital thermometer and record subsequent temperature checks in postnatal record

Hypothermia

- Although babies are able to maintain stable body temperature, their ability to stay warm may be overwhelmed by extremes of environmental temperatures and influenced by gestational age

- A newborn is more likely to develop hypothermia because of large surface area per unit of body weight

> *Close observation by healthcare providers can often prevent neonatal hypothermia*

Temperature <36.4°C in an otherwise well baby

- Apply hat to prevent further heat loss

- Encourage continued skin-to-skin contact with covering blanket

- Initiate early feeding

- Observe for general wellbeing

- Recheck temperature within 1 hour

- If temperature remains <36.4°C, consider heated cot and further investigations – follow local protocol

Temperature ≥38°C

> *Temperature ≥38°C is abnormal and requires urgent attention.*
> *Notify neonatology team who will undertake full assessment, including physical examination*

- If baby appears unwell, or not maintaining own temperature, refer to neonatologist

- If problems identified, continue to observe baby until resolved. Document all management in postnatal records including discussions with parents

HYPOGLYCAEMIA

- Unless unwell, babies do not become hypoglycaemic even if feeding is delayed

- keep warm and encourage to feed as soon as possible. They will suck well, settle between feeds and will not require monitoring – see **Hypoglycaemia** guideline in the Staffordshire, Shropshire & Black Country Newborn and Maternity Network Neonatal guidelines (if used locally)

Symptoms and signs

- Signs of hypoglycaemia may require further investigation including possible admission to neonatal unit

- Blood glucose <2.6 mmol/L and any of the following symptoms:

- apnoeic/cyanotic episodes
- irritability
- hypotonia
- poor responsiveness
- seizures

Management

- See **Hypoglycaemia** guideline in the Staffordshire, Shropshire & Black Country Newborn and Maternity Network Neonatal guidelines (if used locally)

INITIAL CARE AND FIRST EXAMINATION BY MIDWIFE

First hour of birth

- If baby appears unwell or has symptoms of hypoglycaemia, attempt to feed and refer to neonatology team

- Explain feeding cues to mother and offer help initiating first feed (see **Breastfeeding** guideline in the Staffordshire, Shropshire & Black Country Newborn and Maternity Network Neonatal guidelines (if used locally)

- Document first feed in intrapartum record, include:

- feeding method
- time feed started
- duration of feed

Issue 3
Issued: April 2015
Expires: April 2017

- If problems identified, continue to observe until resolved and document management in postnatal record – including discussions with parents
- Once skin-to-skin contact ceased, further assess newborn. Include:
- birth weight
- head circumference
- initial examination
- Document all findings and discussions in intrapartum record

EXAMINATION

- To Identify major physical abnormalities/problems

Consent and preparation

- Inform parents and obtain consent
- Keep baby warm and examine in quiet environment – ideally with parents present

Procedure

Skin

- Hydration
- Rashes: including erythema toxicum, milia, miliaria, *staphylococcal* skin infection, candida
- Colour: pink/cyanosis/jaundice/pallor/plethora
- Acrocyanosis
- Cutis marmorata
- Bruises: traumatic lesions, petechiae

Head

- Palpate skull for:
- sutures and fontanelle
- excessive moulding or tension of fontanelle

Eyes

- Open gently
- Confirm presence
- Exclude subconjuctival haemorrhage

Ears

- Canal patency
- Position in relation to level of eyes
- tags or pits

Nose

- Patent nares
- Accessory skin tags

Mouth

- Use torch to check:
- palate intact
- signs of 'tongue-tie' (defined by NICE as an inability to extend the tongue beyond tip of lower incisors)
- presence of any teeth

Neck

- Run fingers down neck towards trunk to check for abnormal swelling or webbing

Arms and legs

- Extend and check for:
- position, including talipes, symmetry of movement and muscle tone
- exclude trauma during delivery e.g. swelling, fractures and bruising
- presence/absence of digits and webbing of fingers and toes

Hands

- Palmar creases – may indicate congenital abnormality
- Fingers – extra or absent digits and webbing

Back

- Place baby on his/her side or abdomen
- Run fingers downwards along spine to exclude spina bifida or curvature

Chest

- With baby supine, check presence of nipples and normal chest movement

- look for abnormal breathing e.g. flaring of nostrils, sub or intercostal recession, grunting, raised respiratory rate. If present, seek neonatal review

Anus

- Presence and normality of appearance and position

Cord stump

- Examine to confirm presence of 3 vessels. If only 2 identified, neonatal junior doctor must review and document

External genitalia (to determine sex)

Male

- Gently examine scrotum with thumb and forefinger. Check for descended testes and note any hydrocele

- Penis – check position of urethra and exclude hypospadias

Female

- Separate labia to confirm presence of vaginal and urethral orifices

- Examine perineum to detect sinuses

If evidence of ambiguous genitalia, avoid gender assignment before expert evaluation to avoid confirmation of wrong sex.

Ask consultant neonatologist to discuss with parents as soon as possible.

Always use the term 'baby' and avoid using 'he', 'she' or, most importantly, 'it'

Abnormalities

- If baby unwell e.g. respiratory distress or has a major abnormality e.g. spina bifida, inform neonatal team immediately

- note other minor abnormalities and inform neonatal team next working day for prompt referral to appropriate clinician e.g. medical, surgical, orthopaedic etc

- If abnormalities (or deviations from the norm) detected, inform parents and record findings and discussion in intrapartum record

- If in doubt, discuss with delivery suite co-ordinator immediately

- If community birth, community midwife will arrange admission to hospital for mother and baby

VITAMIN K

Prophylaxis

- Vitamin K (Konakion MM Paediatric) as a single dose (see **Table** overleaf for dosage schedule)

- avoid IV administration for prophylaxis as it does not provide the same sustained protection as IM

- See **Vitamin K** guideline in Staffordshire, Shropshire & Black Country Newborn and Maternity Network Neonatal guidelines

Issue 3
Issued: April 2015
Expires: April 2017

Prophylaxis dosage

	Konakion MM Paediatric
Healthy babies of ≥36 weeks	**First line** ● 1 mg IM at birth or soon after **Second line** ● 2 mg oral at birth, then ● 2 mg oral at 4–7 days, then ● 2 mg oral at 1 month if exclusively breastfed
Term babies at special risk ● Instrumental delivery, caesarean section ● Maternal treatment with enzyme-inducing anticonvulsants (carbamazepine, phenobarbital, phenytoin), rifampicin or warfarin ● Requiring admission to NICU ● Babies with cholestatic disease where oral absorption likely to be impaired	1 mg IM at birth or soon after **Do not** offer oral vitamin K
Preterm babies <36 weeks but ≥2500 g	1 mg IM at birth or soon after
All babies <2500 g	400 microgram/kg (0.04 mL/kg) IM shortly after birth (maximum dose 1 mg) Do not exceed this parenteral dose The frequency of further doses should depend on coagulation status
Babies who have or may have Factor VIII or Factor IX deficiency or other coagulation deficiency	Give orally unless results of Factor assays normal

Babies with birth weight ≥2500 g

● Administer Konakion MM Paediatric 1 mg (0.1 mL) intramuscularly

● this is approximately **half** the ampoule volume and should be drawn up using 0.5 mL Omnican-F syringe with 0.01 mL graduations supplied with ampoule

Babies with birth weight <2500 g

● Administer 400 microgram/kg (0.04 mL) with a maximum of 1 mg (0.1 mL) of Konakion MM Paediatric intramuscularly

● round up dose to nearest hundredth [e.g. 300 microgram (0.03 mL), 500 microgram (0.05 mL) etc]

● draw up dose using a 0.5 mL Omnican-F syringe with 0.01 mL graduations supplied with ampoule

REGISTRATION AND IDENTIFICATION

Registration

- Register birth – follow local birth registration procedure

Identification

- For the purposes of this guideline, the term 'wristband' will cover wristbands and any other form of identity band
- If wristbands produced by a non-regulated person (e.g. maternity care assistant), they must be counter-checked by a registered professional
- To reduce risk of mis-labelling, **do not** prepare wristbands before delivery
- If used locally, apply security tag to baby as soon as possible

Before applying wristbands

- Check information on wristbands with mother and/or her birth partner

Mother

- Mother's wristband must contain the following information:
- last name
- first name
- date of birth
- NHS number (if not available, use local hospital number until NHS number available)
- allergy information – according to local practice

Baby

- As soon as possible after delivery secure two wristbands to baby. These must contain the following information:
- mother's last name
- baby's date of birth
- time of birth

- baby's NHS number (if not available, use local hospital number until NHS number available)
- if applicable, twin/triplet I/II/III
- Wristbands may cause damage to premature baby's skin – ensure an alternative method of identification is used
- Electronic security tag (if used locally)

Transferring baby

- Before transfer to ward, neonatal intensive care unit (NICU) or other specialist unit, ensure baby has correct identification
- When baby being transferred home, mother and midwife check both identification bracelets

Checking wristbands

- Check daily
- ensure bands *in situ* as per local practice

Detached wristband

- Apply new wristband
- If both wristbands lost:
- inform midwife in charge of shift
- check wristbands of all other babies on ward before replacing
- complete incident report
- If two or more babies do not have wristband, follow local practice for identification

Issue 3
Issued: April 2015
Expires: April 2017

Use this guideline for antenatal and postnatal collapse

CAUSES

- Haemorrhage – see **Antepartum haemorrhage** and **Postpartum haemorrhage** guidelines
- Pulmonary embolus
- Concealed haemorrhage (e.g. broad ligament haematoma, hepatic rupture)
- Amniotic fluid embolus
- Myocardial infarction
- Aortic dissection
- Peripartum cardiomyopathy
- Rheumatic mitral stenosis
- Sepsis
- Intracranial haemorrhage
- Total spinal block (see **Epidural analgesia** guideline)
- Local anaesthetic or magnesium toxicity
- Hypoglycaemia
- Eclampsia (see **Eclampsia** guideline and **Severe pre-eclampsia** guideline)
- Anaphylaxis (follow local guideline for anaphylaxis)

CARDIAC OR RESPIRATORY ARREST

*If a cardiac or respiratory arrest has occurred, call cardiac arrest team and commence cardiopulmonary resuscitation – see **Collapse** algorithm at end of this guideline*

Organise

- Clearly state location of woman
- Crash-bleep resident anaesthetist, junior doctor and middle grade obstetrician (ST3–7 or equivalent e.g. staff grade, clinical fellow)
- Inform consultant obstetrician
- If antenatal arrest after 22 weeks' gestation, call neonatal team
- Ensure arrest team can gain immediate access to maternity unit

- Station someone (e.g. healthcare assistant, student etc) at delivery suite door, to open door and direct team to woman
- Collect cardiac arrest trolleys and defibrillator

Woman

- Avoid aortocaval compression after 20 weeks' gestation
- Manually displace the uterus. Do not consider the baby in this emergency
- An anaesthetist should protect the airway as soon as possible with a cuffed endotracheal tube
- If resuscitative attempts to revive >20 week pregnant woman have failed after 4 min, perform an immediate caesarean section to improve the chances of successful maternal resuscitation. Do this wherever the arrest has occurred without further preparation as she will need to deliver within minutes and there will not be time for preparation or transfer to theatre
- Caesarean section is of no benefit to women <20 weeks' gestation

SUDDEN COLLAPSE

Woman

- Avoid aortocaval compression after 20 weeks' gestation
- tilt the woman at least 30° using a wedged resuscitation board or a wedge, or manually displace uterus
- Check A, B and C and give oxygen at maximum rate via face mask

Organise

- Bleep consultant obstetrician, on-call obstetric anaesthetist, junior doctor and middle grade obstetrician (ST3–7 or equivalent e.g. staff grade, clinical fellow) – follow local practice

- Summon as many staff as possible and allocate specific tasks, e.g:
- taking observations
- recording events and their management, with times
- communication
- runner for samples and equipment
- support for family

Observations

- Commence HDU chart and observe:
- pulse
- blood pressure – at least every 15 min
- respiratory rate
- pulse oximetry
- If possible, transfer woman to room where HDU care can be provided

Investigations

- Check capillary blood glucose using BM stick
- Insert at least one large IV cannula
- Take blood for:
- FBC
- clotting studies including fibrin degradation products
- crossmatch 2 units of blood
- blood cultures
- U&Es and glucose
- LFTs
- Troponin T or Troponin I [(whichever is used locally) (a marker for myocardial infarction)]

> *It is the responsibility of person obtaining sample to complete blood bottles and forms*
> *Send bloods urgently to laboratory with healthcare assistant or porter*
> *Phone laboratory to request results urgently*

- Obtain arterial blood gases and consider arterial line insertion
- Arrange portable chest X-ray, particularly if oxygen saturation reduced or central venous catheter inserted owing to risk of pneumothorax
- 12-lead ECG – particularly important if any form of cardiac disease suspected
- ECG must be reviewed by a doctor competent in ECG interpretation

History and examination

- Obtain history from those present before collapse occurred
- Examine woman to try to identify most likely cause of collapse

IV access and fluids

- Commence IV fluids
- Unless cardiopulmonary function is rapidly restored, consider a central venous catheter

FURTHER TREATMENT

● Further treatment is dependent on diagnosis

Diagnosis	Treatment
Pulmonary embolism	See **VTE – Pulmonary embolism** guideline
Concealed haemorrhage	See **Antepartum haemorrhage** and **Postpartum haemorrhage** guidelines
Amniotic fluid embolism	See **Amniotic fluid embolism** below
Myocardial infarction	Seek advice from cardiologist
Aortic dissection	
Peripartum cardiomyopathy	
Rheumatic mitral stenosis	
Sepsis	See **Sepsis** guideline
Intracranial haemorrhage	Seek advice from physician
Total spinal block	Call consultant anaesthetist – See **Epidural analgesia** guideline
Toxicity	Call consultant anaesthetist – See **Epidural** guideline, **Eclampsia** guideline or **Severe** eclampsia guideline
Hypoglycaemia	IV glucose – see **Diabetes** guidelines
Eclampsia	See **Eclampsia** guideline
Anaphylaxis	Give adrenaline 500 microgram (0.5 mL of 1:1000 solution) **IM** into midpoint of anterolateral aspect of thigh

Be aware of increase in cardiac causes of collapse

Risk factors for myocardial infarction

● Obesity

● Pre-existing hypertension

● Diabetes mellitus

● Family history

● Age >35 yr

Symptoms and signs prompting investigation

● Severe chest pain

● Chest pain radiating to neck, jaw or back

● Chest pain associated with other features (e.g. agitation, vomiting or breathlessness, tachycardia, tachypnoea and orthopnoea)

Aortic dissection is a cause of chest or intrascapular chest pain, particularly in the presence of systolic hypertension. It is commonly associated with Marfan's syndrome. If suspected, request urgent cardiologist review

AMNIOTIC FLUID EMBOLISM

● Rare and often fatal

● Presentation usually sudden during labour or immediately postpartum

● Acute dyspnoea, cyanosis, shock, cardiac arrest, bleeding from disseminated intravascular coagulation (DIC) and tonic-clonic seizures may all occur

● Sudden change in woman's behaviour can be an early warning feature

TREATMENT

As above, plus:

- If necessary, deliver immediately – ideally vaginally. If not possible, by caesarean section under general anaesthetic

- Insert second large bore (16 G) IV cannula and prepare to manage massive obstetric haemorrhage (see **Postpartum haemorrhage** guideline)

- Consider early insertion of central venous catheter and arterial line

- Discuss need for blood products (including fresh frozen plasma to correct DIC) with consultant haematologist, without waiting for blood results

- Woman will require circulatory support, which can include inotropes, with invasive monitoring

- Transfer to Critical Care Unit

- Report all cases of suspected or proven amniotic fluid embolism, whether fatal or not to National amniotic fluid embolism register via UKOSS (UK obstetric surveillance system)

Issue 3
Issued: April 2015
Expires: April 2017

Maternal collapse algorithm

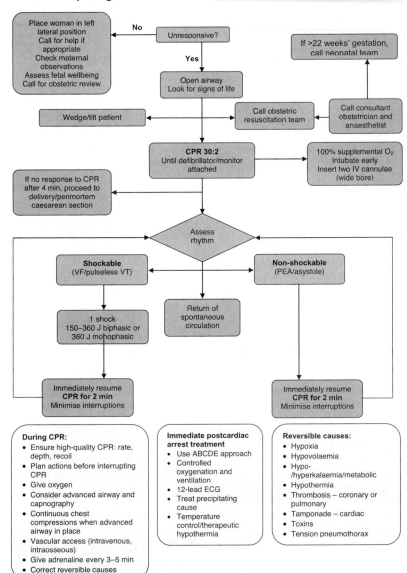

During CPR:
- Ensure high-quality CPR: rate, depth, recoil
- Plan actions before interrupting CPR
- Give oxygen
- Consider advanced airway and capnography
- Continuous chest compressions when advanced airway in place
- Vascular access (intravenous, intraosseous)
- Give adrenaline every 3–5 min
- Correct reversible causes

Immediate postcardiac arrest treatment
- Use ABCDE approach
- Controlled oxygenation and ventilation
- 12-lead ECG
- Treat precipitating cause
- Temperature control/therapeutic hypothermia

Reversible causes:
- Hypoxia
- Hypovolaemia
- Hypo-/hyperkalaemia/metabolic
- Hypothermia
- Thrombosis – coronary or pulmonary
- Tamponade – cardiac
- Toxins
- Tension pneumothorax

See also:

- **Labour management** guideline
- **Latent phase of labour** guideline

DELAY IN FIRST STAGE

- Cervical dilatation <2 cm in 4 hr in first labours
- Cervical dilatation <2 cm in 4 hr, or slowing in progress of labour for second or subsequent labours

Assessment of progress

- Include:
- parity
- rate of cervical dilatation
- woman's emotional state
- descent and rotation of baby's head
- changes in strength, duration and frequency of uterine contractions

Interventions

- Give support, hydration and appropriate and effective pain relief

Amniotomy

- Advise this will shorten labour by approximately 1 hr but may increase strength and pain of contractions
- Two hours after amniotomy, perform vaginal examination. Delay confirmed if cervix has dilated <1 cm
- Amniotomy alone is not an indication for electronic fetal monitoring (EFM)

Oxytocin

- Once diagnosis of delay made by vaginal examination 2 hr after amniotomy, consider oxytocin – see **Oxytocin** guideline
- in a nulliparous woman, midwife may start oxytocin after discussion with obstetric team

> *Before commencing oxytocin, middle grade obstetrician (ST3–7 or equivalent e.g. staff grade, clinical fellow) must review parous woman.*
> *If previous caesarean section, discuss use of oxytocin with obstetric consultant.*
> *Perform at least an abdominal palpation*
> *Repeat vaginal examination may also be appropriate*

- Advise woman that oxytocin will increase frequency and strength of contractions and, where anaesthetist available, offer epidural before oxytocin started
- commence EFM

Monitoring

- Perform vaginal examination 4 hr after commencing oxytocin
- if at least 2 cm progress, repeat vaginal examination 4-hrly
- if <2 cm progress after 4 hr of regular contractions, further review by obstetric medical team and possible caesarean section

SECOND STAGE

Definition

Passive second stage

- Full dilatation of cervix without involuntary, expulsive contractions

Active second stage

- Vertex or breech visible
- Expulsive contractions
- Active maternal effort in absence of expulsive contractions

DELAY IN SECOND STAGE

Definition of delay

Nulliparous women

- Active second stage is delayed if baby not delivered after 2 hr

Parous women

(Includes multipara women who have had previous caesarean section)

- Active second stage is delayed if baby not delivered after 1 hr

Assessment of progress

- Include:
- maternal behaviour
- effectiveness of pushing
- fetal wellbeing
- fetal position and station
- These factors help determine timing of vaginal examinations and need for middle grade obstetrician (ST3–7 or equivalent e.g. staff grade, clinical fellow) review

Management

All women

- In nulliparous women with inadequate contractions at **start** of second stage, consider oxytocin with epidural
- If woman excessively distressed, support, sensitive encouragement and adequate analgesia are particularly important
- Continue epidural top-ups in second stage
- Change position
- Ensure bladder empty
- Perform amniotomy
- If contractions adequate, there is no advantage to starting oxytocin

Women who have received an epidural

- Following diagnosis of full dilatation, delay active pushing (active second stage) for 1 hr unless:
- head visible
- woman has urge to push
- concern about fetal wellbeing
- Oxytocin is not routinely required in second stage

Nulliparous women

- Allow up to 1 hr passive second stage (with or without epidural)
- Then, after 1 hr of active second stage, perform a repeat vaginal examination to assess progress and perform amniotomy, if membranes still intact. Inform midwife co-ordinator
- in absence of any progress, consider asking middle grade obstetrician (ST3–7 or equivalent e.g. staff grade, clinical fellow) to expedite delivery
- If delivery not occurred in a nulliparous women within 2 hr of start of active second stage, call middle grade obstetrician (ST3–7 or equivalent e.g. staff grade, clinical fellow). See **Timing of delivery** below

Parous women

- Allow up to 1 hr passive second stage (with or without epidural)
- After 1 hr of active second stage, call middle grade obstetrician (ST3–7 or equivalent e.g. staff grade, clinical fellow) – see **Timing of delivery** below

Monitoring

- Review advancement of presenting part every 15–30 min until delivery

TIMING OF DELIVERY

- Delivery should occur within 3 hr for a nulliparous and within 2 hr for a parous woman of the active second stage

> *The time taken to perform a caesarean section or instrumental delivery (especially if a trial in theatre indicated) must be taken into account when timing decision for operative delivery*

Issue 3
Issued: April 2015
Expires: April 2017

BACKGROUND

- Approximately 2–5% of births in England and Wales involve women with diabetes

- Approximately 87.5% of pregnancies complicated by diabetes are due to gestational diabetes, with 7.5% due to Type 1 and the remaining 5% to Type 2 diabetes

Pre-existing diabetes

Type 1

- Pancreatic islet beta-cell destruction

- Increased risk of maternal diabetic ketoacidosis

- Characterised by:

- absolute insulin deficiency

- abrupt onset of severe symptoms

- dependence on exogenous insulin to sustain life

Type 2

- Defects in insulin secretion, almost always from insulin resistance

- May be asymptomatic and remain undiagnosed

Gestational diabetes

- Defined as carbohydrate intolerance of variable severity with onset of first recognition during pregnancy

PREGNANCY CONFIRMED

Drugs

- Folic acid supplements 5 mg/day from preconception at least until 12 weeks' gestation

- Aspirin 75 mg/day for pre-gestational diabetes from 12 weeks' gestation

- Review medications

- metformin can be prescribed in pre-conception period, during pregnancy and breastfeeding and can be used as an adjunct to insulin

- stop any angiotensin converting enzyme inhibitor (ACEI) medication and angiotensin receptor blocker (ARBs) and start methyldopa or labetalol as an alternative for hypertension

- beta blockers can mask signs of hypoglycaemia

- stop statins

- Refer women with diabetes or previous gestational diabetes to diabetic antenatal clinic as soon as pregnancy diagnosed. See **Care in diabetic antenatal clinic** overleaf

- If woman has had gestational diabetes in previous pregnancy, offer early self-monitoring of blood glucose or OGTT at 16–18 weeks. If first test result normal, further OGTT at 24–28 weeks

Table 1: Risks from diabetes

To mother	To fetus
• Miscarriage	• Congenital malformation
• Hypoglycaemia/hyperglycaemia	• Stillbirth/neonatal death
• Ketoacidosis	• Premature delivery
• Hypertension/pre-eclampsia	• Fetal macrosomia
• Retinopathy/nephropathy	• Birth trauma
• Induction of labour/caesarean section	• Neonatal hypoglycaemia
• Future diabetes	• Polycythaemia
	• Future obesity and diabetes

Issue 3
Issued: April 2015
Expires: April 2017

CARE IN DIABETIC ANTENATAL CLINIC

● Women with confirmed diabetes to have contact with diabetes team every 2 weeks for assessment of glycaemic control

● timing of contact will depend on local policy and woman's individual needs

Table 2 – Antenatal care (joint obstetric/diabetic clinic)

Appointment	Care of women with diabetes during pregnancy
6–9 weeks	● Confirm viability and gestational age by ultrasound scan ● Information, advice and support on glycaemic control, establish extent of complications ● Refer to dietitian for dietary assessment and advice ● Review medications ● Retinal and renal assessment if not in previous 12 months
Booking appointment (10 weeks)	● Advice about how diabetes will affect pregnancy, birth and early parenting
16 weeks	● Review glycaemic control ● HbA_{1c} levels, retinal (and renal) assessment if required
18–20+6 weeks	● Anomaly scan (including four chamber view of fetal heart and outflow tracts)
24 weeks	● Routine antenatal care
28 weeks	● Ultrasound monitoring of fetal growth and amniotic fluid volume ● Retinal assessment (as required) for women with pre-existing diabetes who did not have diabetic retinopathy at their first antenatal clinic visit
32 weeks	● Ultrasound monitoring of fetal growth and amniotic fluid volume
36 weeks	● Ultrasound monitoring of fetal growth and amniotic fluid volume ● Plan delivery – see **Diabetes – Labour** guideline ● timing ● mode of delivery ● analgesia/anaesthesia ● therapy during and after birth ● care of baby/breastfeeding
38–39 weeks	● Induction of labour/caesarean section
40 weeks	● If well controlled gestational diabetic on diet, can wait until 40 weeks

Management of diabetes

Monitor blood glucose targets

- Advise women to test fasting and 1-hour postprandial blood glucose levels after every meal during pregnancy
- Aim for fasting blood glucose of 3.5–5.9 mmol/L and 1-hour postprandial blood glucose <7.8 mmol/L

Treatment

- In most women, gestational diabetes will respond to changes in diet
- if diet and exercise do not control blood glucose levels and if ultrasound shows incipient fetal macrosomia, give metformin and/or insulin
- In Type 1 and 2 diabetes, adjust therapy to maintain blood glucose targets

> **Metformin and insulin are the only diabetes medications safe for use in pregnancy**

Women on insulin

- Discuss risks of hypoglycaemia
- offer concentrated oral glucose solution to women taking insulin, and glucagons to women with type 1 diabetes. If accepted, train woman and partner to use
- Discuss risk of diabetic ketoacidosis

DIABETIC KETOACIDOSIS

- Diabetic ketoacidosis is a medical emergency
- inform both obstetric and medical consultants and manage woman in a high dependency setting
- stabilisation of DKA may be necessary before considering emergency delivery

Issue 3
Issued: April 2015
Expires: April 2017

PREPARATION

- Discuss with woman

Time and mode of delivery

- Woman with diet-controlled or metformin controlled diabetes with normally grown fetus:
- advise induction of labour not to be delayed beyond 40 weeks' gestation
- Woman on insulin:
- advise induction of labour at 38 weeks' gestation
- Woman on insulin pump:
- manage as per local Trust policy

Analgesia and anaesthesia

- Offer women with diabetes and co-morbidities (e.g. obesity or autonomic neuropathy) obstetric anaesthetic assessment in third trimester

Care during and after labour

- Analgesia and anaesthesia
- Good glycaemic control
- Continuous fetal monitoring
- Prevention of neonatal hypoglycaemia
- Care of baby/breastfeeding

PRETERM LABOUR

- Pulmonary maturation delayed in fetuses of diabetic women, particularly where control has been poor
- Where premature delivery anticipated for women with confirmed diabetes, give betamethasone– see **Preterm labour** guideline
- Steroid administration worsens diabetic control and may lead to ketoacidosis in women with pre-existing type 1 diabetes – anticipate an increase in insulin requirement and administer using your local variable rate IV insulin infusion VRIII (sliding scale) regimen

INDUCTION OF LABOUR

- See **Induction of labour** guideline

Diabetic control

- Before labour established, normal metformin/insulin regimen and diet, together with blood glucose monitoring

DURING LABOUR

Risk

- Increased risk of shoulder dystocia particularly if baby macrosomic – ensure middle grade obstetrician (ST3–7 or equivalent e.g. staff grade, clinical fellow) is available on delivery suite during second stage – see **Shoulder dystocia** guideline
- Increased risk of cephalopelvic disproportion – be vigilant for delay and, if occurring, use oxytocin with caution

Monitoring during labour

Woman

- Record capillary glucose level hourly
- Once VRIII regimen commenced, monitor blood glucose hourly
- Monitor blood glucose at 30 min intervals after induction of general anaesthesia and birth of baby until woman fully conscious
- Test all urine samples for ketones
- if positive, refer to local policy for management of diabetic ketoacidosis

Continuous fetal monitoring

- Maternal hyperglycaemia may cause fetal acidosis. If any EFM abnormalities, check maternal glucose
- Fetal blood sampling if indicated, as normal labour – see **Fetal blood sampling** guideline

Metformin and diet controlled

- If blood glucose elevated e.g. persistently above local Trust policy threshold, commence insulin and IV fluid regimen **below**
- When labour established, stop metformin

Gestational diabetes mellitus

- **Insulin controlled** – Dependent upon amount of insulin required – dosage as per local Trust policy

Elective caesarean section

- If caesarean section carried out before 39 weeks' gestation, consider administration of antenatal steroids with a VRIII (sliding scale regimen). Refer to local Trust guideline for management
- Women on insulin:
- admit as in-patient the night before procedure
- Commence insulin and fluid regimen (if required), following local policy

Emergency caesarean section

- Check blood glucose level and commence insulin and IV fluid regimen **below**

INSULIN AND IV FLUID REGIMEN

- 500 mL glucose 10% with 10 mmol potassium chloride 8-hrly
- 50 units soluble insulin (Actrapid/ Humulin S) in 50 mL sodium chloride 0.9% via syringe pump according to blood glucose checked at time of admission and hourly thereafter by glucometer
- Determine rate of fluid infusion depending on blood glucose concentration and local policy
- Aim to keep woman's blood glucose concentration between 4–9 mmol/L

- Most women will need 2–4 units/hr
- Avoid large changes in insulin infusion rate and therefore in glucose concentration
- If blood glucose not maintained within normal range, contact diabetes team

> *Always use commercially produced pre-mixed bags of glucose 10% with potassium*

POSTNATAL MANAGEMENT

- Diabetes team will write management plan

> *Inform women with insulin-treated diabetes that they are at increased risk of hypoglycaemia in postnatal period, especially when breastfeeding. Advise to have a meal or snack available before or during feeds*

Stopping insulin and fluid regimen

- Continue VRIII regimen until able to eat and drink normally

Type 1 diabetes

- Revert to pre-pregnancy insulin requirements or the regimen advised by diabetes team
- Keep VRIII running for 30–60 min after first subcutaneous insulin dosage
- May require less insulin if planning to breastfeed
- Review by diabetes team as appropriate

Type 2 diabetes

- Stop insulin and fluid regimen
- Postnatal regime as planned with diabetes team. Review blood glucose
- Metformin not contraindicated in breastfeeding, but avoid sulphonylureas

Issue 3
Issued: April 2015
Expires: April 2017

Gestational diabetes

- Women with gestational diabetes mellitus will cease all diabetic treatment after delivery
- Arrange postnatal GTT or fasting blood glucose at 6 weeks according to local Trust policy

Neonatal care

- See Staffordshire, Shropshire & Black Country Newborn and Maternity Network Neonatal **Hypoglycaemia** guideline or follow local practice

FUTURE PLANS/ PRE-PREGNANCY ADVICE

For women with pre-existing and previous gestational diabetes

Planning next pregnancy

- Discuss importance of planned pregnancy and role of contraception

Lifestyle

- Stop smoking and alcohol
- Increase exercise

Diet

- Well distributed carbohydrate intake – Provide information on carbohydrate counting/food portion sizes
- Good range of low glycaemic index foods especially fruit and vegetables
- Moderate fat intake
- Awareness of current safe foods during pregnancy www.nhs.uk/livewell/pregnancy/pages/healthyeating.aspx
- Consider referral to dietitian for individualised dietary advice

Ideal body weight

- If BMI >27, offer advice on weight-loss before conception

For women with pre-existing diabetes

- **All the above, plus:**

Glycaemic control

- Explain that good glycaemic control before conception and throughout pregnancy will reduce risk of miscarriage, congenital malformation, stillbirth and neonatal death
- Optimise diabetic control (e.g.HbA_{1c} <6.1%). May need to switch to insulin to obtain this
- Advise women with HbA_{1c} >10% to avoid pregnancy

Screen for complications

- Retinal and renal assessment

Drugs

- Folic acid supplements 5 mg/day from preconception until 12 weeks' gestation
- Aspirin 75 mg/day for pre-gestational diabetes from 12 weeks' gestation
- Review medications
- metformin can be prescribed in the pre-conception period, during pregnancy and breastfeeding and can be used as an adjunct to insulin
- stop any angiotensin converting enzyme inhibitor (ACEI) medication and angiotensin receptor blocker (ARB) and start methyldopa or labetalol as an alternative for hypertension
- beta blockers can mask signs of hypoglycaemia
- stop statins

INDICATIONS FOR WHO AND WHEN TO SCREEN

Early screening	24–28 weeks
• If gestational diabetes in a previous pregnancy, offer early self-monitoring of blood glucose or oral glucose tolerance test (OGTT) at 16–18 weeks. If result normal, further OGTT at 28 weeks	• BMI >30 kg/m^2 • Previous macrosomic baby ≥4.5 kg • Previous gestational diabetes • First degree relative with Type 1 or Type 2 diabetes • Family origin with a high prevalence of diabetes – south Asian, black Caribbean and middle Eastern • Previous unexplained stillbirth

How

- Use 2 hr 75 g OGTT to test for gestational diabetes
- Screen positive
- fasting plasma venous glucose concentration ≥5.6 mmol/L or
- 2 hr plasma venous glucose concentrations ≥7.8 mmol/L
- See **Diabetes – Antenatal care** guideline

INTRODUCTION

- DFM may identify at-risk fetuses
- The evidence that intervention can improve the outcome is less convincing

RECOGNITION

- Woman reports DFM, often by phone
- If ≤24 weeks' gestation, arrange midwife to see her within 24 hr in hospital or community
- If >24 weeks' gestation, advise woman to attend maternity department

MANAGEMENT

Assessment at any gestation

- Check for previous or current medical problems (e.g. bleeding, oligohydramnios, polyhydramnios, small for dates, pre-eclampsia, hypertension, diabetes mellitus)
- Blood pressure
- Urinalysis
- Abdominal palpation to assess fetal growth
  - plot on fetal growth chart

Investigations

- If fundus small for dates against fetal growth chart:
  - ultrasound scan for growth, liquor volume
  - umbilical artery Doppler study
- Electronic fetal monitoring (EFM) trace dependent on gestation – see below
  - EFM trace is a test for hypoxia. When used in the antenatal period, it is essentially an assessment of immediate fetal condition

≤24 weeks' gestation

- Auscultate fetal heart, separately identifying maternal pulse

- If normal assessment:
  - reassure woman that irregular movement patterns can be experienced in early pregnancy
  - advise to return again if concerned about fetal movements
- Manage any abnormalities found

24–26 weeks' gestation

- Auscultate fetal heart and assess symphysis fundal height
- If normal assessment:
  - reassure
  - resume normal antenatal care
  - advise her to return if further concerns about movements
- If reduced symphyis fundal height, refer for obstetric assessment

Second episode of DFM

- Growth scan (unless performed in previous 2 weeks)

26–28 weeks' gestation

- **Perform EFM trace**, ideally computerised (if available)
- **Criteria met within 45 min:** reassure, allow home and advise to return if further concerns about fetal movements
- **EFM trace suspicious or pathological:**
  - inform middle grade obstetrician (ST3–7 or equivalent e.g. staff grade, clinical fellow) urgently
  - consider cannulation
  - FBC and group and save
  - consider transfer to delivery suite
- **Criteria not met after 45 min:** continue EFM and call middle grade obstetrician (ST3–7 or equivalent e.g. staff grade, clinical fellow)
- If symphysis fundal height reduced for dates, arrange growth scan (unless performed in previous 2 weeks)

- If adequate EFM trace cannot be obtained despite midwife sitting with woman, seek middle grade obstetrician (ST3–7 or equivalent e.g. staff grade, clinical fellow) opinion

>28 weeks' gestation

First episode DFM

- EFM trace, ideally computerised (if available)
- Assess symphysis fundal height
- if symphysis fundal height reduced for dates, arrange growth scan (unless performed in previous 2 weeks)
- **EFM trace normal with fetal movement felt and no risk of fetal growth restriction (FGR)/stillbirth identified:**
- reassure, allow home and advise to return again if concerned about fetal movements
- **EFM trace normal with persistent DFM and/or risk factor for fetal growth restriction (FGR)/stillbirth identified:**
- reassure, allow home and advise to return again if concerned about fetal movements and expect to be contacted for a growth scan
- arrange growth scan (unless performed in previous 2 weeks)
- manage any abnormalities found
- **EFM trace suspicious or pathological:**
- inform middle grade obstetrician (ST3–7 or equivalent e.g. staff grade, clinical fellow) urgently
- consider cannulation
- FBC and group and save
- transfer to delivery suite

Second episode DFM

- EFM trace, ideally computerised (if available)

- **EFM trace normal:**
- reassure, allow home and advise to return again if concerned about fetal movements and expect to be contacted for a growth scan
- arrange growth scan (unless performed in previous 2 weeks), liquor volume and umbilical artery Doppler
- After 28 weeks' gestation, women with second episode of DFM within one month of first DFM:
- refer to their consultant's next antenatal clinic
- **EFM trace suspicious or abnormal:**
- inform middle grade obstetrician (ST3–7 or equivalent e.g. staff grade, clinical fellow) urgently
- FBC and group and save
- consider cannulation
- transfer to delivery suite

Management plan in labour

- Continuous EFM in labour
- If admitted with ruptured membranes or suspected early labour, EFM

EFM TRACE AND DFM SUSPICIOUS/PATHOLOGICAL

- **EFM trace suspicious/pathological:**
- inform middle grade obstetrician (ST3–7 or equivalent e.g. staff grade, clinical fellow) urgently
- FBC and group and save
- All women with suspicious/ pathological EFM must be reviewed by middle grade obstetrician (ST3–7 or equivalent e.g. staff grade, clinical fellow). It may or may not be appropriate to repeat EFM. If repeated, consider computerised EFM if available

> *Remember EFM is an investigation. Continuing the monitoring will not improve fetal condition – use whole clinical picture to assess fetal wellbeing*

Issue 3
Issued: April 2015
Expires: April 2017

- If an appropriately repeated EFM trace is normal, it may be reasonable to allow woman home

- Arrange growth scan to exclude other cause for concern about fetal wellbeing, (e.g. reduced liquor), which might also predispose to decelerations from cord compression

INABILITY TO IDENTIFY FETAL HEART

- Ultrasound scan (ideally in maternity scan department)

- If out-of-hours, performed by middle grade obstetrician (ST3–7 or equivalent e.g. staff grade, clinical fellow) or consultant competent to use portable labour ward ultrasound machine

- If scan identifies fetal death (second trained operator to confirm this), inform on-call consultant obstetrician. It is unlikely that woman will need immediate delivery – see **Fetal loss** guideline

Eclamptic seizures are often self-limiting. See also – **Severe pre-eclampsia** guideline

RESUSCITATION AND STABILISATION

- **A**irway, **B**reathing **C**irculation and lateral tilt

- Do not leave woman alone. Call for help from senior midwife, senior obstetrician and inform consultant obstetrician and consultant anaesthetist to attend as soon as possible

- During convulsion, consider personal safety and aim to prevent maternal injury

- as soon as possible, position woman in recovery position and administer 15 L oxygen via close-fitting face mask

- Attach pulse oximeter and automatic blood pressure monitor

- As soon as is **safely** possible, site two 16 gauge (grey) Venflons

- Insert Foley indwelling catheter, and monitor urine output hourly with strict fluid restriction

INVESTIGATIONS

- Obtain blood and send urgently for:

- FBC

- clotting studies

- U&E

- LFT

- urates

- group and save

- Consider arterial blood gases

TREATMENT

- Magnesium sulphate is treatment of choice – See **Severe pre-eclampsia** guideline, **Magnesium sulphate**

- Treat recurrent seizures with either further IV bolus of magnesium sulphate or increase in infusion rate – See **Severe pre-eclampsia** guideline, **Magnesium sulphate**

- If repeated seizures not responding to magnesium sulphate, consultant obstetrician and anaesthetist decide on use of diazepam 5–10 mg or thiopentone, together with intubation and transfer to intensive care. Consider CT scan to exclude other causes

- Blood pressure control – see **Severe pre-eclampsia** guideline

Post seizure

- Once seizure ended, auscultate lungs and commence continuous oxygen saturation monitoring

- Transfer to an area where high dependency care can be provided

- Full neurological assessment following seizure to rule out localising signs of alternative causes e.g. intra-cranial haemorrhage

- Once woman stabilised, plan to deliver

- Monitor conscious level and document on HDU chart

Delivery

- See **Severe pre-eclampsia** guideline

> *Eclampsia is nearly always an indication for rapid delivery regardless of gestation*
> *Woman's condition will always take priority over fetal condition*

POSTNATAL CARE

- HDU care for minimum of first 24 hr as for severe pre-eclampsia

- Subsequent postnatal management – See **Severe pre-eclampsia** guideline

- Record incident using local incident reporting procedure

Drugs

- See **Severe pre-eclampsia** guideline

Issue 3
Issued: April 2015
Expires: April 2017

AIM

Recognition and prevention of potential adverse outcomes to at risk fetuses

ANTENATAL MONITORING

Indications for EFM

Maternal

- Pre-eclampsia/eclampsia
- Antepartum haemorrhage
- Prolonged ruptured of membranes >24 hr
- Prolonged pregnancy >42 weeks
- Induced labour
- Abdominal pain
- Trauma/after a fall/RTA
- Cholestasis
- Abnormality on auscultation (abnormal baseline, decelerations)

Fetal

- Intrauterine growth restriction/abnormal Doppler
- Preterm labour
- Oligohydramnios/polyhydramnios
- External cephalic version
- Iso-immunisation
- Suspicious antenatal EFM trace
- Reduced fetal movements >26 weeks' gestation

When to monitor

- >26 weeks' gestation

How to monitor

- Perform abdominal examination
- Listen to fetal heart (FH) with a Pinard stethoscope before commencing EFM
- Palpate maternal pulse simultaneously to differentiate fetal and maternal heart rates

Duration of monitoring

- Until reactivity observed – usually 10–40 min
- two accelerations in 10 min is a reactive trace. Sleep pattern with no acceleration does not exceed 40 min in vast majority
- Document reasons for monitoring >40 min in maternal healthcare record

INTERPRETATIONS AND ACTIONS

Normal/reassuring

- Normal EFM has four reassuring features:
- baseline 110–160 beats/min
- baseline variability >5 and not >25 beats/min
- accelerations present
- no decelerations

Action

- Repeat according to clinical situation and degree of fetal risk

Non-reassuring features

- Baseline 161–170 beats/min or 100–109 beats/min
- Accelerations absent
- Reduced variability <5 beats/min for >40 min
- Any deceleration
- Sinusoidal pattern (oscillation frequency <2–5 cycles/min, depth 2–10 beats/min for >40 min with no area of normal baseline variability)

Action

- Arrange review by middle grade obstetrician (ST3–7 or equivalent e.g. staff grade, clinical fellow) and decide if delivery indicated; if in doubt, discuss with consultant obstetrician
- Consider ultrasound scan for fetal growth
- Babies can also be compromised from other causes e.g. sepsis, anaemia

Dawes and Redman fetal heart rate (FHR) variation assessment (if local practice)

- Assessment of FHR variation requires computerised analysis, given the large inter and intra individual variation when assessed visually
- Consider gestational age, recording duration and clinical indication

Abnormal

- STV <4 ms
- Absence of high frequency episodes

Action

- Arrange review by middle grade obstetrician (ST3–7 or equivalent e.g. staff grade, clinical fellow) as above

> **Do not keep repeating a non-reassuring EFM. Decide if delivery is indicated.**
> **If necessary, consultant obstetrician to review EFM**

INTRAPARTUM MONITORING

Indications for EFM

Maternal

- Oxytocin augmentation
- Epidural anaesthesia
- Vaginal bleeding
- Maternal pyrexia 38°C once or 37.5°C twice 2 hr apart
- Previous caesarean section/uterine rupture
- Hypertension
- Pregnancy post term (>42 weeks)
- Prolonged membrane rupture interval (>24 hr)
- Induced labour where more than a single dose of prostaglandin has been required
- Diabetes
- Antepartum haemorrhage
- Maternal medical disease that may increase risk to fetus e.g. significant cardiac disease, renal disease. If unsure, discuss with middle grade obstetrician

- Antiphospholipid antibody syndrome
- Recurrent miscarriage (three consecutive miscarriages)
- Obstetric cholestasis
- Previous stillbirth

Fetal

- Meconium stained liquor (see **Meconium stained liquor** guideline)
- Abnormal FHR on auscultation:
  - baseline abnormality <110 beats/min >160 beats/min, decelerations after a contraction
- Fetal growth restriction
- Prematurity (<37 weeks' gestation)
- Oligohydramnios
- Polyhydramnios
- Abnormal Doppler artery studies
- Multiple pregnancy
- Breech presentation
- Two episodes of reduced fetal movements in a one month period after 28 weeks' gestation
- Any woman who has had a suspicious or pathological EFM trace antenatally especially if performed for reduced fetal movements

Frequency of assessment

- Undertake a systematic assessment every hour to categorise FHR trace based on classification in **Tables**
  - document findings as per local practice

INTERPRETATIONS AND ACTIONS

Inadequate quality

- Check maternal pulse
- Check position of transducer of fetal scalp electrode
- Unless contraindicated (e.g. prematurity, hepatitis B or C), consider applying fetal scalp electrode

Classification

Table 1: Categories and definition of FHR traces [NICE clinical guideline 55 (2007)]

Category	Definition
Normal	All 4 features are classified as reassuring
Suspicious	One feature is non-reassuring
Pathological	≥2 non-reassuring features or ≥1 abnormal feature

Table 2: Classification of fetal heart rate features [NICE clinical guideline 55 (2007)]

Feature	Baseline (beats/min)	Variability (beats/min)	Deceleration	Acceleration
Reassuring	110–160	≥5	None	Present
Non-reassuring	100–109 161–180	<5 for 40–90 min	Typical variable decelerations with over 50% of contractions, for >90 min Single prolonged deceleration up to 3 min	Absence of accelerations with an otherwise normal EFM trace is of uncertain significance
Abnormal	<100 >180 sinusoidal pattern ≥10 min	<5 for 90 min	Either atypical variable decelerations with over 50% of contractions or late decelerations, both for over 30 min Single prolonged deceleration for >3 min	

- If repeated accelerations present with reduced variability, regard FHR trace as normal
- True early uniform decelerations are rare and benign, and not significant
- Most decelerations in labour are variable
- An increase in heart rate even within normal range, with other non-reassuring or abnormal features should increase concern
- If FHR trace to date considered normal, short breaks may be allowable up to 15 min for personal care (toilet, shower). Such interruptions should be infrequent and should not be immediately after any intervention that might be expected to alter FHR e.g. amniotomy

Suspicious category of FHR

General

- Report to midwife in charge or middle grade obstetrician/consultant
- Consider digital stimulation of fetal scalp during vaginal examination as an adjunct to EFM

Identify any reversible causes

- Initiate appropriate actions immediately to improve fetal condition:
- maternal repositioning or turning to left lateral position to alleviate hypotension or cord compression
- check blood pressure, especially if after an epidural top-up, and correct hypotension
- review oxytocin infusion rate and continue. To achieve satisfactory contractions (4 or 5 in 10 min) increase rate. To alleviate contraction related fetal compromise, reduce rate
- Correct dehydration
- Treat maternal pyrexia

Pathological category of FHR

- Report to midwife in charge/middle grade obstetrician/consultant
- middle grade obstetrician or consultant to carry out full assessment
- Stop oxytocin infusion until reviewed by middle grade obstetrician or consultant

- Correct reversible causes as above
- Use tocolytics for hyperstimulation
- subcutaneous terbutaline 250 microgram
- Undertake fetal blood sampling for pathological EFM trace where appropriate/feasible along with conservative measures to improve fetal condition See **Fetal blood sampling** guideline
- When making decision about fetal wellbeing, consider time taken for delivery

> *If no recovery of pathological EFM trace with correction of reversible causes, consider fetal blood sampling. Urgent delivery may be indicated*

Fetal bradycardia >3 min

- Urgent medical review and prepare to urgently expedite delivery. If bradycardia not recovered by 9 min, prepare and transfer woman to theatre
- if FHR recovers and maintains at normal baseline, obtain woman's and consultant's opinion and reconsider decision for delivery

RECORDING AND DOCUMENTATION (intrapartum and antenatal monitoring)

- **Machine** – set speed 1 cm/min, set date and time, ensure identification, ensure adequate quality of FHR and uterine contraction recordings and improve quality with necessary adjustment
- if there are artefacts, change machine
- ensure setting in multiple pregnancy
- Ensure the following are recorded on EFM trace:
- date, time and signature of midwife at commencement of trace

- **maternal** – label name, hospital number, pulse rate, date and time
- **fetal** – auscultation
- **events** – note any events on trace during monitoring e.g vaginal examination, FBS
- **opinion** – add comment on EFM trace e.g. 'normal', 'suspicious', 'pathological' with date time and signature
- **completion** – sign again, enter name, date, time and mode of delivery
- **Storage** – follow local practice for storing trace
- Document plan in maternal healthcare record
- Hourly use of 'fresh eyes' is best practice

MATERNAL REFUSAL TO BE MONITORED

- A woman can refuse monitoring. Respect her wishes and offer discussion with senior staff
- Explain risks and benefits and, in the event of refusal, monitor baby by auscultation which, if in baby's best interest, may lead to intervention for delivery
- Clearly document maternal refusal, discussion and explanation of risks and benefits in maternal healthcare record

Issue 3
Issued: April 2015
Expires: April 2017

INTRODUCTION

Epidural analgesia is the most effective method of pain relief in labour. Discuss the following benefits with the mother:

- Reduced neonatal respiratory depression (repeat doses of IM opioids)
- Improved uteroplacental blood flow in the compromised fetus
- Assists with controlled birth (e.g., breech or multiple pregnancy)
- If epidural analgesia is available on a 24 hr basis, time from informing anaesthetist until he/she is able to attend should ideally not exceed 30 min

If delay anticipated

- Review necessity of epidural: purely analgesic or medical indication
- If only for analgesia, midwife to discuss alternative form of pain relief with the woman until epidural service is available
- Document 'exceptional circumstances', cause of delay and discussion with woman in maternal healthcare record. Involve on-call consultant anaesthetist in the discussion

INDICATIONS

- Maternal request
- Obstetric indications (pre-eclampsia, breech, multiple pregnancies, prolonged labour)
- Medical indication (CVS and respiratory diseases, etc)
- Morbid obesity

CONTRAINDICATIONS

Absolute

- Patient refusal
- Local or systemic sepsis
- Known hypersensitivity to local anaesthetic drugs
- Coagulopathy – see **Investigations**
- Raised intracranial pressure
- Inadequately trained or competency assessed staff

Anticoagulant therapy

- Do not insert epidural:
  - for at least 12 hr after last prophylactic dose
  - for at least 24 hr after last therapeutic dose

Relative

Discuss with consultant obstetric anaesthetist

- Neurological disorders (spinal bifida occulta)
- Significant cardiac disease
- Anatomical deformity or back surgery
- Haemorrhage, hypovolaemia

PREPARATION

Patient

- Explain technique, and risks and benefits
- Provide information leaflet (if available locally)
- Obtain and document verbal consent
- Obtain IV access

Investigations

- In pre-eclamptic women, check FBC. If platelet count <100,000 – APPT, INR
- Intra-uterine death >1 week: detailed coagulation profile including D-dimer and fibrinogen levels
- In septic woman: FBC and CRP

Equipment

- Oxygen and suction available
- Epidural trolley with:
  - epidural pack (16 G/18 G Tuohy needle) or 19 G/23 G catheter
  - yellow epidural infusion lines labelled with yellow label from pack
  - sterile gown, gloves, hat and mask
  - chlorhexidine skin preparation 0.5%
- Use specific epidural pumps with locking ability

Optional equipment

- CSE pack/spinal needles 25 G

Drugs

- Lidocaine 1%

- Standard mixture (bupivacaine 0.1% with fentanyl 2 microgram/mL) or a bag of 0.1% bupivacaine and fentanyl ampoule for mixture preparation

- Levobupivacaine (0.25 and 0.5%) (for bolus administration in second stage of labour)

- Vasopressors

- Sodium chloride 0.9%

INSERTION OF EPIDURAL

- Use full aseptic technique wearing gloves, gown, hat and mask

- Clean insertion site with alcoholic chlorhexidine gluconate solution and allow to **air dry**

- Evidence suggests that loss of resistance to sodium chloride 0.9% is a better technique than loss of resistance to air

- If technical difficulty, seek help early or consider alternative analgesia e.g. remifentanil PCA

ESTABLISHING AND MAINTAINING EPIDURAL ANALGESIA

Accepted regimens

1. Continuous infusion

2. Patient controlled epidural analgesia (PCEA)

3. Bolus administration PRN

Drug used for all three procedures

- Mixtures of low concentration of local anaesthetic (e.g. bupivacaine 0.1% or levobupivacaine) with an opiate (e.g. fentanyl 2 microgram/mL), as per local Trust protocol

Test dose for all epidural procedures

- Administer a test dose of 5 mL from the epidural solution

- Wait for five min to check for rapid onset of sensory changes and significant decrease in blood pressure

Procedures for establishing analgesia in labour

1. Procedure for continuous infusion of dilute mix of local anaesthetic and opioid

- After verification of correct catheter placement, administer loading dose (usually 10–15 mL of the mixture), then:

- commence an infusion rate of 10–12 mL/hr for maintenance

- rate may be increased up to 15 mL/hr and rescue analgesia may be provided by a single bolus of 10 mL of the infusion mixture. Can be administered by midwife via pump

2. Procedure for use of PCEA

- Anaesthetist will set up the machine

- Administer the first 10 mL bolus dose of mixture

- Set patient administered bolus of 10 mL infusion. Set a bolus lockout of 24 min

- Commence a background infusion rate of 0–5 mL/hr of the mixture

- **Do not give** first patient administered dose before 30 min after first therapeutic dose

- **Do not give PCEA handset to woman until 30 min after infusion commenced**

- if pain relief remains ineffective after two boluses, request duty anaesthetist to assess woman

Issue 3
Issued: April 2015
Expires: April 2017

3. Procedure for bolus epidural top-up

- Anaesthetist will administer first bolus dose of epidural (10–15 mL of the drug mixture) after the test dose
- Subsequent boluses are 10 mL of mixture administered by either midwife or anaesthetist

Top-up by midwife

- Midwife will check each prescribed top-up (10 mL of drug mixture) with another qualified professional before administering. Following administration, both will sign and record on regional anaesthesia chart or as per Trust policy

INTRAPARTUM CARE

- **Monitor:**
- pulse, blood pressure, respiratory rate, sensory, motor block and conscious level – as per local practice
- Maintain venous access for as long as epidural analgesia is maintained
- Continuous electronic fetal monitoring when receiving epidural blockade throughout labour

> *If there are concerns for fetal wellbeing at any stage, abandon the procedure until a proper assessment of fetal status is made*

Positioning

- To reduce the risk of hypotension, do not allow woman to lie flat on her back. For pressure care encourage her to change position regularly

Mobility

- Assess ability to ambulate 20–30 min after initial injection:
- ability to raise each leg from bed for at least 5 sec
- ask if she feels capable of weight-bearing

Before weight-bearing

- Other requirements to be satisfied include:
- no postural hypotension
- co-operative woman
- A partner and/or midwife must be available at all times to accompany woman while mobilising

Bladder care

- Epidural analgesia may make passing urine difficult and woman may not be aware of a full bladder. Encourage her to void her bladder every 2–4 hr

Diet and fluids

- Acceptable drinks include water, tea, coffee, squash and non-fizzy isotonic sports glucose
- Oral ranitidine 150 mg every 6–8 hr while in labour

Epidural management during second and third stage of labour

- Do not withhold epidural analgesia in second stage
- Usual dose for second stage of labour is 10 mL levobupivacaine 0.25% via epidural catheter. Do not leave woman unattended for 20–30 min after bolus
- Maintain epidural analgesia until perineal suturing has been performed

An anaesthetist must give top-ups in the following situations

- Midwife is concerned about level of block
- An unusual prescription has been ordered
- A hypotensive episode (systolic blood pressure <100 mmHg) after previous top-up
- Analgesia is persistently inadequate
- To extend the block for caesarean section
- After suspected dural tap and with intrathecal catheter *in situ*

HIGH CONCENTRATION TOP-UPS

Caution: This type of epidural top-up has a higher rate of hypotension, significant intravascular injection, difficulty in pushing and instrumental delivery

Indications

- Has a role in managing inadequate analgesia, premature desire to push and instrumental delivery

Administration

- Requires levobupivacaine 0.25% or lidocaine 2% (dose dependent on circumstances and anaesthetist assessment)
- Care for woman on bed and encourage to change position regularly

EPIDURAL CATHETER REMOVAL

- **Do not** remove for at least 12 hr after prophylactic and 24 hr of therapeutic LMWH administration
- In severe PET and after a massive bleed, ensure normal FBC and clotting profile before removal
- Unless otherwise directed by anaesthetist, remove just before discharge back to ward
- Pull firmly on catheter, but **do not** use excessive force – catheter should come out easily with minimal resistance
- Remove catheter and check blue tip is complete
- Document removal of catheter and whether tip intact
- Inform anaesthetist of any problems

TRANSFER BACK TO WARD

- Before transferring to ward, midwife should:
- ensure vital signs are normal
- adequate return of motor power to legs and document – if not, contact anaesthetist

COMPLICATIONS AND MANAGEMENT

Total spinal and unanticipated high block

- Can occur after first dose of epidural or any time during labour
- Monitor as per local protocol

It is an acute emergency, characterised by:

- Rapidly progressive sensory and motor block of legs and arms
- Severe hypotension and bradycardia
- Reduced or absent respiration
- Altered level of consciousness

Management

- Call for help – including an anaesthetist
- Relieve aortocaval compression by left lateral displacement of the uterus – manually or with a wedge
- If CPR not required, full lateral position
- Use ABC approach
- Administer 100% oxygen and, if respiration inadequate or woman has lost consciousness, be ready to intubate
- Cardiovascular support in the form of fluids, vasopressors (phenylephrine, ephedrine, adrenaline)
- In case of cardiac arrest or severe cardiac depression, initiate CPR – see **Maternal collapse algorithm in Collapse** guideline
- If no return of spontaneous circulation, consider peri-mortem caesarean section within five min
- After successful resuscitation, woman must be managed by on-call consultant anaesthetist (if not already there)

Incomplete block

- Check – has the catheter fallen out?
- Is there a leak/disconnection?
- Try bolus of standard mix or stronger solution as indicated

Issue 3
Issued: April 2015
Expires: April 2017

Unilateral block

- Anaesthetist may consider pulling catheter back 1–2 cm and try another dose with the painful side dependent. Optimum is 3–4 cm of catheter in epidural space

- If still not effective, consider resiting epidural

Missed segment, patchy block

- Try using 5 mL levobupivacaine 0.25%

- If block patchy and high, consider possibility of a subdural block – see **Accidental dural puncture** overleaf

- If still not effective, consider resiting epidural

Perineal pain

- Give bolus of 10 mL infusion mixture

- If pain persists, try topping up with 50–100 microgram fentanyl in 8–10 mL levobupivacaine 0.25%

- If inadequate analgesia after bolus, anaesthetist to review

Breakthrough pain through a good block

- Consider uterine rupture or abruption

- Assess woman and progress of labour

> *If inadequate analgesia after 1 or 2 top-ups and woman still unhappy, anaesthetist to review in person, resite or seek senior help*

Pruritus

- If of sufficient severity to warrant treatment, administer one dose of naloxone 40 microgram IV

- Alternatively, consider chlorpheniramine (Piriton) 4 mg oral or 10 mg IM

- If concern about traumatic or bloody tap, consider deferring next LMWH dose

Intravascular injection of local anaesthesia

- Arises as a result of incorrect site of administration (IV) or incorrect dose administered

Symptoms and signs

- Peri-oral numbness, difficulty speaking

- Tinnitus

- Dizziness

- Restlessness

- Dysrhythmia (bradycardia, VT and VF)

- Hypotension

- Convulsions

- Loss of consciousness

Immediate management

- **Stop injecting drug**

- Commence resuscitation, all principles of basic and advanced life support apply

- Summon help immediately including anaesthetist if not present

- If lateral tilt of 15–30 degrees cannot be applied, manually displace uterus

- Give benzodiazepine, thiopental or propofol in small incremental doses to control seizures

- Bag-mask ventilate with 100% oxygen before intubation

- Perform caesarean section

Use of 20% intralipid

- Early use of 20% intralipid IV 1.5 mL/kg over 1 min, followed by an infusion of 15 mL/kg/hr

- **After five min,** give **maximum of two** repeat boluses (same dose) if:

- CVS stability is not achieved or adequate circulation deteriorates

- Leave **five** min between boluses

- a maximum of **three** boluses can be given (including the initial bolus). followed by infusion dose to 30 mL/kg/hr

- Continue infusion until stable and adequate circulation restored or maximum dose of lipid emulsion given
- Recovery after a cardiac arrest will take >1 hr
- Consider drawing blood for analysis

> ***Do not exceed a maximum cumulative intralipid dose of 12 mL/kg***

Accidental dural tap

- Incidence of dural puncture whilst siting an epidural is 1–2%
- Overall incidence of post dural puncture headache (PDPH) following inadvertent dural puncture is 75%

If recognised at time of insertion

- Leave catheter intrathecally for at least 24 hr or re-site
- Label clearly as a spinal/intrathecal catheter
- Give 1 mL bupivacaine 0.25% with fentanyl 25 microgram. Alternatively, use 2 mL of the infusion mixture. Flush with 2 mL sodium chloride 0.9% after every top-up
- Subsequent boluses must be 2 mL of the infusion mixture administered by anaesthetist only

Monitor

- Regular BP (timing according to local practice)
- Keep vasopressors handy
- Keep woman on labour ward until catheter removed

> ***If intrathecal catheter placement difficult, seek senior help or provide alternative methods of analgesia e.g. remifentanil PCA***

Follow-up after dural puncture

- Anaesthetist to discuss dural puncture with woman
  - assess for symptoms of PDPH and treatment options available with attendant risks and benefits
- Provide information leaflet (if available locally)
- Ensure details recorded in audit book or according to local practice

DEFINITION

A surgical incision of the perineum to increase the diameter of the vulval outlet during childbirth to facilitate delivery but minimise harm to mother and baby

Perform mediolateral episiotomy only

Mediolateral episiotomy

● Cut starts at centre of the vaginal fourchette and is directed to the right side at an angle of 60 degrees to the vertical axis (see diagram)

INDICATIONS

The list below is not exhaustive – use clinical judgement on an individual basis

● Fetal distress

● Maternal reason to expedite delivery (e.g. pre-eclampsia/eclampsia)

● Rigid perineum preventing delivery

● Instrumental delivery (particularly forceps)

● Occipitoposterior position (OP)

● Shoulder dystocia

● Breech presentation

Equipment

● Sterile or tap water to clean area before procedure

● 1 x 10 mL syringe

● 1 x 22 gauge (green) infiltration needle

● 10 mL lidocaine 1%

● Mayo episiotomy scissors

Consent

● Reassure woman and partner

● Explain procedure and indications

● Obtain and record consent

PROCEDURE

This procedure must only be performed by appropriately trained practitioners or under direct supervision of a mentor

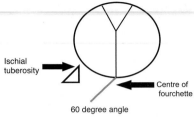

Ischial tuberosity

Centre of fourchette

60 degree angle

Anus

Position and preparation of women

● Place in comfortable legs-open position

● Cleanse perineal area using aseptic technique

● Place index and middle fingers into vagina between presenting part and perineum

● Insert needle fully into perineal tissue starting at centre of fourchette and direct it midway between ischial tuberosity and anus (protect fetal head)

● Draw back plunger of syringe before injecting 5–10 mL lidocaine 1% slowly as needle is withdrawn

Episiotomy incision

● Insert middle and index fingers into vagina and gently pull perineum away from fetal part to protect fetal head

● Perform incision when presenting part has distended perineum

● Insert open scissors between two fingers and make incision in one single straight cut to minimise damage and allow/facilitate optimal realignment

● begin at the centre of the fourchette and extend 4 cm in a right mediolateral direction midway between the ischial tuberosity and anus, ideally at a 60 degree angle to vertical axis

● Withdraw scissors carefully

● Control delivery of the presenting part and shoulders to avoid extension

● If delay in delivery, apply pressure to episiotomy between contractions to control bleeding

● After third stage, thoroughly inspect vagina/perineum to ascertain extent of trauma

COMPLICATIONS

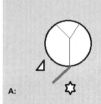

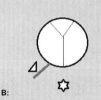

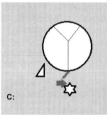

Figure A	Figure B	Figure C
Correct anatomical position	**Incorrect** ● Cut begins lateral to the centre of the fourchette ● Will not increase diameter of vulval outlet ● Will cause damage to bartholins gland ● Will affect lubrication and may cause complications e.g. dyspareunia	**Incorrect** ● Cut is too small resulting in extension of incision towards the anus and increasing risk of anal sphincter injury

Suturing

See **Third and fourth degree tears** guideline and **Perineal trauma suturing (tears and episiotomy)** guideline

Pain management

See **Perineal trauma (tears and episiotomy)** guideline

Discharge and follow-up

See **Perineal trauma (tears and episiotomy)** guideline

Issue 3
Issued: April 2015
Expires: April 2017

INTRODUCTION

- Management of babies born at the threshold of viability presents some of the most testing ethical and clinical problems
- If it seems likely that delivery will occur at an extremely premature gestation, there may be a variable amount of time to counsel and prepare woman and partner for the outcome
- Unless circumstances dictate otherwise, senior staff should always be involved
- Document all information given to parents in the maternal healthcare record

Table 1

Gestation	Senior neonatologist to counsel	Neonatal middle grade * or consultant at delivery	Electronic fetal monitoring	Caesarean section (CS) indicated	CS indicated if breech/ non-cephalic
<22 weeks	No	No	No	Not for fetal indications	No
22–22+6 weeks	Yes, if parents request	No	No	Not for fetal indications	No
23–23+6 weeks	Yes	Yes	No	Not for fetal indications	No
24–24+6 weeks	Yes Parents visit NNU if possible	Yes	Fetal heart auscultated 2nd stage	Not for fetal indications	No
25–25+6 weeks	Yes Parents visit NNU if possible	Yes	Yes	*May* be justifiable for fetal indications	No
26–26+6 weeks	Yes Parents visit NNU if possible	Yes	Yes	Indicated for fetal compromise	Uncertain
27–27+6 weeks	Yes Parents visit NNU if possible	Yes	Yes	Indicated for fetal compromise	Uncertain
28 weeks	Yes Parents visit NNU if possible	Yes	Yes	Indicated for fetal compromise	Advise CS

* ST3–7 or equivalent e.g. staff grade, clinical fellow

> *These are guidelines only*
> *An alternative management plan, based on individual circumstances,*
> *can be made by a senior obstetrician*
> *Record management plan clearly in maternal healthcare record and*
> *ensure it is accessible to all staff*

OBSTETRIC RESPONSIBILITIES

Calculating gestational age

- Management of extreme prematurity depends on gestation. Knowledge of precise gestation is important, preferably calculated from an ultrasound scan at 9–14 weeks

- Dating scans are accurate within one week below 14 weeks. However, even at 20 weeks they are accurate to within one-and-a-half weeks

- If only late ultrasound scan is available, use best estimate gestation to determine management

- If estimated gestation is ≥23 weeks and fetal heart is audible before delivery, a neonatologist experienced in resuscitation to attend birth

Counselling

- By senior obstetrician, who will provide patient information leaflet (if available). Ask the following questions:
- how sick is baby now
- how sick is baby likely to be at birth
- is baby likely to die or survive
- Use EPICure data (see **Tables 2 and 3**)
- Discuss the role of operative delivery (risks and benefits) and the use of fetal monitoring with woman and family and take their views into account

Electronic fetal monitoring (EFM)

- Perform EFM **only** if it has been agreed with parents after discussion that an emergency caesarean section would be performed for a pathological EFM

- It is often difficult to monitor a fetus <29 weeks' gestation

- If an adequate trace cannot be obtained, baby's wellbeing is not being monitored

- As a minimum, a senior obstetrician must discuss with parents whether to deliver or continue labour without monitoring

- Document discussion and decision in maternal healthcare record

Antenatal steroids

- Decision to give betamethasone to improve fetal lung maturity <24 weeks' gestation must be discussed with consultant obstetrician

MAGNESIUM SULPHATE

- Magnesium sulphate protects premature babies' brains from cerebral palsy. Consider for all babies <30 weeks' gestation likely to deliver in next 24 hr regardless of mode of delivery

- Can be given to women with multiple pregnancy and irrespective of whether steroids have been given

- ideally, commence infusion 4 hr before delivery but there may still be benefit if given <4 hr before delivery but do not delay delivery in time-critical situations e.g. fetal distress

- administration may be impractical when delivery is imminent. Consultant obstetrician will decide whether to administer

Side effects

- Inform woman about the possibility of side effects. The most common are:
- facial flushing
- nausea and vomiting
- sweating
- Tachycardia and hypotension have also been observed
- The effect may be more pronounced when magnesium sulphate is given with calcium channel blockers e.g. nifedipine

Issue 3
Issued: April 2015
Expires: April 2017

Dosage

- Give loading dose of 4 g (8 mL) IV over 20 min

- mix 4 g (8 mL) magnesium sulphate 50% with 12 mL sodium chloride 0.9% (total 20 mL) and set syringe driver at 60 mL/hr

- Give maintenance dose of 1 g/hr IV via syringe pump until delivery or for 24 hr whichever is sooner

- mix 5 g (10 mL) magnesium sulphate 50% with 40 mL sodium chloride 0.9% (total 50 mL) and set syringe driver at 10 mL/hr

- If woman did not deliver as expected, a repeat dose can be given later in the pregnancy

Observations and monitoring

- Commence hourly observations of:

- respiratory rate

- level of consciousness

- Check deep tendon reflexes regularly (according to local practice). In general, use patella tendon reflexes, use reflexes at elbow or wrist in women who have a working epidural *in situ*

- Check reflexes more often when:

- there is oliguria

- woman is also taking nifedipine

- magnesium sulphate dosage has required adjustment

- Monitor oxygen saturation continuously with a pulse oximeter. Stop infusion immediately and call middle grade obstetrician (ST3–7 or equivalent e.g. staff grade, clinical fellow) if:

- tendon reflexes absent

- respirations <12/min

- SpO_2 <96%

- abnormal conscious level

- urine output <1.5 mL/kg over 4 hr

Antidote

- 1 g (10 mL 10% solution) calcium gluconate IV over 3 min

NEONATAL RESPONSIBILITIES

- Wherever possible, inform neonatal team of woman's admission to delivery suite

- If appropriate, neonatologist will review woman and discuss care of baby following delivery

- Counselling provided by a senior neonatologist, depending on gestation (see **Table 1**), should include the role of resuscitation, use of cardiac drugs and risks and benefits

- Use EPICure research study data to give a percentage for survival and risk of disability (see **Tables 1** and **2**). Local data may also be useful

Neonatal resuscitation

Certain gestation of <22^{+0} weeks

- Advise parents that survival is not possible

Certain gestation of 22^{+0}–22^{+6} weeks

- Advise parents that survival is extremely rare (see EPICure data) and it would be in baby's best interests, and standard practice, not to resuscitate

Certain gestation of 23^{+0}–23^{+6} weeks

- Decision **not** to start resuscitation may be appropriate, particularly if parents have expressed this wish

- If resuscitation is started, initiate mask ventilation and observe heart rate response

- if there is a very rapid improvement, intubation, stabilisation and transfer to NNU is appropriate

- There is no evidence to support the use of chest compression or epinephrine in babies <25 weeks

Certain gestation of 24+0–24+6 weeks

- Unless parents and clinicians have considered baby will be born severely compromised, start resuscitation

- Initiate mask ventilation and observe baby's heart rate. If there is a very rapid improvement, intubate, stabilise and transfer to NNU

- There is no evidence to support the use of chest compressions or epinephrine in babies <25 weeks

Certain gestation of 25+0–25+6 weeks

- Start resuscitation

- Initiate mask ventilation and observe heart rate response. If there is a very rapid improvement, intubate, stabilise and transfer to NNU

- If appropriate, initiate chest compressions and epinephrine – follow NLS guidelines and **Cardiopulmonary resuscitation of the newborn** guideline

Certain gestation of 26+0 weeks and above

- Advise parents that survival at this gestation is usual

- It is considered good practice to offer parents the opportunity to raise questions regarding care of the newborn with a member of the neonatal team. Include a visit to the neonatal unit if feasible

- If complications anticipated e.g. known congenital anomaly, provide counselling by a senior member of the neonatal team (who should document the discussion in the woman's healthcare record)

EPICURE STUDIES OF SURVIVAL AND DISABILITY

Table 2: EPICure 2 study – Survival and disability

Completed weeks of gestation	%	22	23	24	25	26
Survival to discharge as % live births	%	1	15	36	62	75
Survival to discharge as % babies admitted to NICU	%	16	29	46	69	78
Survival without disability at 3 years	%	1	15	36	43	59
Survival without disability of those admitted to NICU	%	5	15	28	47	61

Table 3: Factors affecting chance of survival

Increase	Decrease
Female sex	Prolonged membrane rupture interval
Birth weight 50-85th centile	Sepsis
Birth weight > 600 g	Birth weight <500 g
Delivery in unit with level 3 NICU	Abnormal umbilical artery Doppler flow

Issue 3
Issued: April 2015
Expires: April 2017

COMMUNICATION WITH PARENTS

- Dependent upon labour timescales etc, a second counselling session may be useful

- Following discussion, parents should be aware of the options, their risks, benefits and the implications of alternatives

- Reinforce verbal information by providing printed leaflets (if available). Give details of support services available e.g. bereavement counselling and BLISS information (http://www.bliss.org.uk/order-publications/)

- When talking to parents, survival outcomes may need to be modified in light of clinical information available see **Table 3**

- The RCOG states that 'conveying the concept that fetal death is not the worst outcome, and that severe neonatal morbidity and maternal and fertility morbidity are also important considerations to the woman and her partner, must be conducted with kindness and sensitivity'

- Doctor counselling parents should not impose his/her cultural or religious convictions on those whose beliefs may differ. When a doctor's beliefs prevent the disclosure of all available management options, he/she has a duty to refer woman to a colleague

- If there is a difference of opinion between clinical staff and parents regarding management, seek a second opinion

CERTIFYING NEONATAL DEATH

- Baby must be seen by a doctor while alive (if possible). This does not have to be a neonatologist

- Doctor who saw baby before death issues a medical certificate certifying death. The certificate must always be issued even if baby lived for only a few minutes

- Neonatal death certificates can **only** be issued by a doctor. Midwives do **not** certify neonatal deaths

- When completing the certificate, the doctor prints his/her name after the signature and records their GMC number

- If it is not possible for a doctor to see baby before he/she dies, document this clearly in the healthcare record. Doctor should see baby as soon as possible after death

- In some areas, all deaths must be discussed with the coroner's office. Check your local coroner's requirements before issuing death certificate and requesting post mortem consent

Definition of signs of life

- It is extremely important to distinguish between involuntary, physiological movements and signs of life

- observed movement, such as a jerk of a limb or occasional gasp, are not necessarily signs of life or viability

- in these circumstances, explanations should be given to parents by a senior member of staff and registration as a neonatal death is not necessary

- Where signs of life are evident at birth, inform parents that their baby may continue to show such signs for minutes or even hours following delivery and reassure them that baby will be treated with respect and dignity

- Give parents the opportunity to keep baby with them until he/she dies

- Baby must then be registered as a neonatal death

- Once a baby is born alive he/she acquires the same legal status as any other human being and is owed a duty of care

INTRODUCTION

- Prenatal screening for fetal abnormalities using second trimester ultrasound scan and maternal serum screening is offered routinely in the UK

- Routine second trimester ultrasound scans increase the detection rate for fetal abnormalities compared to scans offered on a selective basis only

- Abnormalities may be detected on an ultrasound scan at any stage of pregnancy

- sensitivity of detection is determined by severity and type of abnormality. More severe abnormalities and those developing earlier have a higher detection rate

- false positive rates from ultrasound scanning are <1%

SECOND TRIMESTER ANOMALY SCANNING

- To identify fetal conditions associated with high morbidity and long-term disability

- Performed between 18–23 weeks' gestation

> *Ultrasound imaging must only be performed by person fully trained in its use and qualified in detection of fetal abnormality using this technique*

Before scan

- Ensure ultrasound equipment is of appropriate standard and in working order

- Check woman's identity

- Inform woman of nature and purpose of the screening proposed and discuss the limitations of ultrasound scanning in detecting fetal abnormality i.e. sensitivity of detection is only 76% even for life-threatening abnormalities

- Treat woman sympathetically and address anxieties or concerns

- If woman does not wish to be informed of any fetal abnormalities, give her the opportunity to decline anomaly scanning but to have a scan to determine placental site and fetal growth

ABNORMALITY DETECTED

- Sonographer performing ultrasound examination must report findings to woman personally

- Inform woman and her partner in descriptive but not diagnostic terms

> *If there is doubt about a diagnosis or a scan feature, refer woman to appropriate expert, giving reason for referral*

Referral

- Within one working day, refer to a consultant obstetrician with fetal medicine expertise

- Fetal medicine consultant will re-scan within 5 days and explain findings to woman and her partner

- it may be necessary to repeat information. Written information and diagrams can be helpful

- When major fetal abnormalities are identified, give parents the Antenatal Results and Choices (ARC) booklet (if used locally)

- It may be appropriate for consultant with expertise in fetal medicine to offer fetal karyotyping by amniocentesis or chorionic villus sampling

- Refer confirmed fetal abnormalities in ongoing pregnancies to neonatologist

- Feticide is recommended for termination of pregnancy after 22 weeks' gestation, which is associated with increased difficulty in managing a woman who elects termination later than this stage

- More complex cases may benefit from referral to a tertiary centre e.g. to obtain access for magnetic resonance (MR) imaging or to receive antenatal counselling from neonatal surgeon

- Complete notification to the regional congenital anomaly register

Normal variants

- It is no longer recommended to screen for 'soft markers for Down's syndrome'. However, the following appearances should be reported and the woman referred for further assessment:
- nuchal fold >6 mm
- ventriculomegaly (atrium >10 mm)
- echogenic bowel (with density equivalent to bone)
- renal pelvic dilatation (AP measurement >7 mm)
- standard growth measurements compared to dating scan (significantly <5th centile on national charts)

Documentation

- A printed formal report must be produced and a copy placed in maternal healthcare record
- Record positive and relevant negative findings that are important to that particular clinical situation
- Store relevant images
- Ensure all reports are dated and signed

SCREENING FOR DOWN'S SYNDROME

- Offer Down's syndrome screening
- combined test (11+2–14+1 weeks) with nuchal scan or quad test (14+2–20 weeks)
- Women with a multiple pregnancy who wish to have Down's screening:
- offer combined test (11+2–14+1 weeks), having had the opportunity to discuss implications of screening in twin pregnancy with either an antenatal screening midwife or fetal medicine midwife – see **Multiple pregnancy** guideline

INVASIVE TESTING FOR FETAL ABNORMALITY

- Performed for fetal karyotyping or other genetic testing

Amniocentesis

- Performed after 15 weeks, by an appropriately trained operator
- rate of miscarriage associated with amniocentesis is approximately 1%

Chorionic villus sampling (CVS)

- Performed after 11 weeks, by an appropriately trained operator
- rate of miscarriage following CVS is approximately 1–2%

BACKGROUND

- Fetal blood sample (FBS) is a sample of blood taken using aseptic technique from the presenting part of the fetus in utero

- Fetal pH can identify fetal hypoxemia and acidosis

- when fetus is hypoxemic, metabolism changes from aerobic to anaerobic, producing lactic acid and a subsequent drop in pH, providing a measure of the degree of hypoxaemia

INDICATIONS

- Consider fetal pH when:

- electronic fetal monitoring (EFM) trace is pathological – see **Electronic fetal monitoring** guideline

- With suspicious EFM, fetal blood sampling can be helpful in planning further management and can be performed in first and second stage of labour

> *Do not undertake FBS where there is clear evidence of acute fetal compromise. Deliver baby urgently.*
>
> *Assess and manage each woman individually and, where there is cause for concern, seek advice from on-call consultant obstetrician*

- Take **two** samples, to ensure reliability of result. Remember a fetal blood sample only reflects the condition of the fetus at the moment of sampling

CONTRAINDICATIONS

- Acute fetal compromise (e.g. unrecovered prolonged deceleration of fetal heart rate >3 min)

- Maternal infection e.g. HIV, hepatitis viruses or herpes simplex virus

- Fetal bleeding disorders e.g. haemophilia

- Prematurity (<34 weeks' gestation)

FBS NOT POSSIBLE

- If FBS necessary but not possible to perform e.g. poor cervical dilatation, woman's refusal, middle grade obstetrician (ST3–7 or equivalent e.g. staff grade, clinical fellow) must seek senior advice from on-call delivery suite consultant obstetrician. Usually, if sufficient concern for a fetal blood sample to be performed, deliver baby urgently

PREPARATION

Equipment

- Sterile FBS pack
- Chlorhexidine acetate BP 0.05% cleansing solution
- Sponge holder
- Amnioscope
- Light source
- Blade
- Blade holder
- Capillary tube pack
- White soft paraffin
- Lubricant gel
- Ethyl chloride spray
- Urinary catheter (if required)
- Fetal scalp electrode (if required)

Consent

- Explain procedure to woman and obtain verbal consent

- document consent in maternal healthcare record

PROCEDURE

> *Take preparation time into consideration when performing repeat samples.*
>
> *If sample result is not available within 30 min, consider need for delivery*

Issue 3
Issued: April 2015
Expires: April 2017

Midwife

- Prepare equipment
- Assistant to (ideally) position woman in left lateral position
- Continue electronic fetal monitoring. If significant deterioration e.g. bradycardia, proceed to urgent delivery
- Inform delivery suite team leader, who will ensure other staff involved (e.g. anaesthetist) are informed
- Avoid leaving woman alone while sample is processed, especially if her legs are on supports

Obstetrician

- Cleanse vulva
- Drape with sterile towel
- Insert lubricated amnioscope to access fetal scalp and connect or position light source
- Clean fetal scalp
- Spray scalp with ethyl chloride spray
- Apply white soft paraffin to area of scalp where FBS sample is to be taken
- Incise scalp with blade, collect sample with capillary tube and give to assistant
- Take a second sample (for immediate analysis in blood gas analyser)
- Clean the area and re-position woman to minimise discomfort

Analysing sample

- A healthcare professional trained in the use of the blood gas analyser will take the samples to the analyser, process the sample and inform obstetrician of result

Umbilical cord samples

- For all deliveries requiring FBS in labour, take paired cord umbilical cord samples at delivery – see **Umbilical cord sampling** guideline

INTERPRETATION OF RESULT

- Interpret all results taking rate of progress of labour and other clinical parameters of woman and baby into account

Result	Action
pH ≥7.25, base excess normal and EFM trace remains pathological	• Repeat samples in **one hour** to ensure fetal pH not deteriorating
pH 7.21–7.24	• Repeat sample in **30 min** (see **Flowchart**) ○ in early high-risk labour, this reading could indicate the need for caesarean section
pH abnormal (e.g. ≤7.2)	• Expedite delivery following discussion with on-call consultant obstetrician

- If EFM trace remains unchanged and a second FBS is stable, further samples may be deferred unless there are additional abnormalities on the EFM trace
- When a third FBS is considered necessary, inform consultant obstetrician
- Interpret results of all repeat samples taking into account the previous result

DOCUMENTATION

- Ensure results sheet is secured in maternal healthcare record and handwritten in intrapartum documentation

Communication

- Ensure parents and family are reassured and fully informed of procedures, individualised plan of care and sequence of events at all times by attending obstetric, neonatal and midwifery staff
- Record all discussions in maternal healthcare record

Flowchart – Fetal blood sampling (FBS) ~ NICE 2007

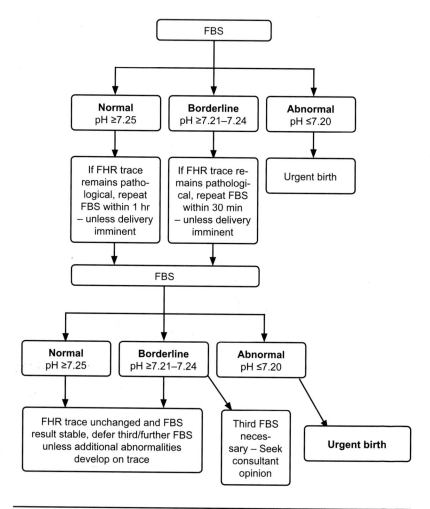

INTRODUCTION

- A parent's relationship with their baby begins long before birth. It is possible to grieve for babies who die before birth, who are born and, for whatever reason, cannot survive and where pregnancy is terminated owing to abnormality

Treat parents and baby with respect, sensitivity and dignity at all times. Inappropriate care can lead to immense dissatisfaction and additional trauma

When a pregnancy ends, for whatever reason, there are a number of common elements and needs in the parents' experience of loss. Some aspects of grief are individual and very private. Aim to support parents and facilitate, as far as is possible, their individual needs

- Required elements of care will depend on circumstances of loss:
- termination of pregnancy for fetal abnormality
- fetal loss <24 weeks' gestation
- stillbirth
- neonatal death
- Complete appropriate local checklist for particular circumstance to ensure no aspect of care is overlooked, even if woman chooses to decline some management options

BEFORE ADMISSION TO DELIVERY SUITE

Diagnosis

- Confirm diagnosis of intrauterine death by ultrasound scan carried out by two qualified and experienced operators
- Arrange review by consultant obstetrician and plan delivery
- Perform observations, MEWS score and record on local documentation
- Unless concerns for woman's safety (e.g. placental abruption, active sepsis), offer the choice to go home and return to delivery suite at a convenient time 24–48 hr later

- provide 24 hr contact number
- Some women will not want to go home and will be admitted soon after being informed of diagnosis of fetal death

Breaking bad news

- Inform parents as soon as anything worrying is suspected even if not yet confirmed or certain
- unless an emergency, provide a woman who is alone the opportunity to call a partner, relative or friend for support and ask if she wishes to wait until they arrive before problem is explained in detail
- If member of staff with parents at the time cannot provide accurate or sufficient information, he/she should inform parents and arrange for a more senior person to see them
- do not give parents inaccurate/ incomplete information that they may later discover is incorrect

Privacy

- Wherever possible, care for woman and family in bereavement suite
- Visiting at woman/parents' request only

Information for parents

- Parents require information at every stage about what is happening, procedures and choices available
- when diagnosis confirmed, gently explain to woman and family the process of induction and time it may take. Written information may be used later to reinforce discussions
- where English is not parents' first language or there is sensory impairment (e.g. deaf/deaf–blind), ensure interpreter available
- Give parents information leaflets available within your Trust

Documentation

Document all discussions with parents in maternal healthcare record

Liaison

- Delivery suite obstetric and midwifery team will liaise with:
- specialist midwife for bereavement (if in post)
- neonatal unit (if appropriate)
- fetal medicine
- antenatal clinic
- chaplaincy
- general office
- community midwives
- GP

DELIVERY

- Discuss with woman the process, analgesia and support that will be offered in labour
- Most women will be advised to have a vaginal birth as it is safer and has less impact on future pregnancies
- For women who have had a previous caesarean section, discuss mode of delivery with consultant obstetrician
- Complete a partogram during labour

Recommended drug regimen

Initial drug dose

- Mifepristone (Mifegyne RU 486) 200 mg oral administered by senior obstetrician on licensed premises. Healthcare professional must observe woman take tablet
- Inform woman of possibility of abdominal discomfort and/or a small amount of bleeding
- reassure that this is normal and regular analgesia, e.g. paracetamol can be taken at home
- Ask woman to remain on premises for one hour to observe side effects
- if vomiting occurs, repeat dose
- Induction may commence at this point or, should the woman wish, she may go home and return 48 hr later
- Provide telephone numbers for delivery suite with instructions to call if she has any concerns while at home

On admission/in labour

- Consultant obstetrician to direct care
- Perform regular maternal observations (see **Labour management** guideline)
- Provide analgesia as required
- if woman requests an epidural, ensure a platelet count is available

Further drug regimen

- No more than 24–72 hr after initial dose of mifepristone 200 mg oral, give misoprostol:
- **<26 weeks' gestation:** 100 microgram vaginally 6-hrly – **maximum 4 doses**
- **>27 weeks' gestation:** 25–50 microgram vaginally 4-hrly – **maximum 6 doses**

> *In previous caesarean section or uterine surgery, where the cavity has been breached (e.g. myomectomy, uterine perforation) use 25–50 microgram dosage*

Side effects of misoprostol

- Pyrexia
- Diarrhoea
- Inform woman she may experience flu-like symptoms
- Particular care is required for women with:
- severe asthma
- previous caesarean section
- CVS insufficiency
- hepatic or renal failure
- adrenal suppression including long-term corticosteroid use

FOLLOWING DELIVERY

Management of third stage

- Give 1 mL syntometrine (oxytocin with ergometrine) IM after delivery
- If woman hypertensive, give oxytocin 10 units IM or 5 mg as a slow IV bolus as an alternative

> *For Rh negative women, obstetrician will prescribe anti-D immunoglobulin*

Lactation suppression

- Provide general advice e.g. wear well-fitting bra
- Offer 1 mg cabergoline for lactation suppression. Contraindicated for hypertensive women

Parent involvement

- If circumstances allow, involve parents in decisions regarding care of their baby
- Give parents the opportunity to see and hold their baby as soon as possible and for as long as they wish. Parents may initially decline to see their baby but should be assured they can change their mind at any time
- They may wish to give their baby a name
- When baby very small, it may be difficult to determine the sex by visual inspection. Where there is any doubt, midwife should not express an opinion even if pressed by parents to do so
- Obtain consent before carrying out any procedure e.g. obtaining mementos, including taking hand and footprints, photographs etc. Include parents in decisions and be guided by their wishes
- Senior obstetrician must see every baby following delivery regardless of gestation and carefully record presence or absence of any visible fetal abnormalities

Religious needs

- Ask parents if they have specific religious beliefs and offer to contact hospital chaplain/faith representative
- Parents may wish to contact their own faith representative

Investigations

- Senior obstetric team member or specialist midwife for bereavement will discuss with parents

Post mortem

- Obtaining consent from parents for post mortem is particularly difficult. Take into account feelings, emotions and religious beliefs of woman, partner and family
- Written consent for examination of a fetus or baby, regardless of gestational age, must be obtained from parent by a healthcare professional competent to take consent for post mortem. Junior medical staff must not seek consent
- Allow time for questions
- Record discussion and consent in maternal healthcare record

Placenta

- Where family requests post mortem, send placenta with baby
- If family do not want a post mortem, send placenta for histology to Birmingham Women's Hospital (if this is local practice)

Cytogenetics

- Indications for cytogenetics
- severe IUGR or known visible fetal abnormality
- Obtain parental consent for cytogenetic investigations or molecular genetic studies of any material from any pregnancy loss regardless of gestation
- request by senior obstetrician and appropriate form signed. This will form evidence of discussion between clinician and parents and of their consent
- unsigned requests will not be processed
- Send to Regional Genetics Laboratory
- if any uncertainty whether test is appropriate, phone the regional genetics laboratory for advice

Additional investigations

Investigation	
• Blood for TORCH (Toxoplasma, rubella, cytomegalovirus and herpes simplex) and parvovirus • High vaginal swab for sexual health screen • Endo-cervical swab for chlamydia	Microbiology
• U&E • LFT • Uric acid • TFT • HbA_{1c} and random glucose • CRP • Bile acids	Clinical biochemistry
• Group and save • Cardiolipin antibodies • Lupus anticoagulant • Thrombophilia screen • Clotting screen • FBC • Kleihauer	Haematology

- For women who have experienced late pregnancy loss, stillbirth or neonatal death, carry out complete local list of blood tests and swabs

- Where pregnancy was medically terminated owing to fetal abnormality, investigations should include at least:

- FBC

- group and save

- swabs (as per local guidance)

CERTIFICATION

- Failure to complete all certification carefully can result in delay registering baby

- Complete stillbirth and neonatal death certificates in black ink

- Print name after signatures and include GMC/PIN number

- Do not use abbreviations

Miscarriage

- For a baby born <24 weeks' gestation showing no signs of life, midwife or doctor present at birth completes local form to allow disposal of fetal remains

Stillbirth

- Doctor or midwife present at birth completes a medical certificate of stillbirth

- A midwife or doctor who has examined the baby after birth can also complete the form but must be certain that the baby was not born alive

Issue 3
Issued: April 2015
Expires: April 2017

Neonatal death

- If baby was born alive, regardless of gestation, a medical certificate for the cause of death in baby dying within the first 28 days of life must be issued

- Medical certificates can **only** be completed by a doctor, neonatologist or obstetrician

- Doctor **must** have seen the baby alive but does not have to have seen the baby after death

Babies born outside hospital without a midwife or doctor present

- Where it is known that intrauterine death occurred before delivery, midwife or doctor examining baby can issue a stillbirth certificate. If there is any doubt, refer to the coroner

- If baby is born alive outside the hospital but has died before arrival at hospital, the coroner must be informed, regardless of gestation

- If parents request a cremation, midwife/doctor completes a cremation certificate

REGISTRATION

- Give family information about how to register their baby. Ensure they have all the required certificates

- There is no legal requirement to register a baby delivered <24 weeks' gestation that shows no signs of life. However, a baby that shows signs of life, whatever gestation, must be registered as a **neonatal death**

- A stillborn child is defined in the Births and Deaths Registration Act 1953 (and amended by Stillbirths Definition Act 1992) as 'any child expelled or issued forth from its mother after the 24th week of pregnancy that did not breathe or show any signs of life', and should be registered as a **stillbirth**

Clarification

- Department of Health and Office for National Statistics have agreed the following under the above Act that:

- if a fetus (or more than one fetus) is expelled after 24 weeks of pregnancy, then, provided it was no longer alive at the 24th week, (this fact being known or provable from the stage of development of the dead fetus) it does not fall within the category of births to be registered as stillbirth(s) under the above Act

- Royal College of Obstetricians and Gynaecologists and Royal College of Midwives have agreed: In a number of situations where it is known that one or more fetuses have died before the 24th week of pregnancy, those fetuses do not have to be registered as stillbirths. For example:

- where there has been a delay between diagnosed intrauterine death and delivery

- vanishing twins or selective or multifetal pregnancy reduction in multiple pregnancies

- fetus papyraceous

- In all cases there must be evidence that it was known that the fetus or fetuses had died before the 24th week of pregnancy. This evidence, usually based on ultrasound imaging, must be clearly detailed in maternal healthcare record for future reference

- Occasionally there is no ultrasound evidence available when one or more fetuses is born dead >24 weeks' gestation. It may be appropriate to use stage of development of the fetus(es) as an indicator of when death occurred relative to the 24th week limit. This must be determined on a case by case basis by an obstetrician of at least middle grade (ST3–7 or equivalent e.g. staff grade, clinical fellow) – it is not the responsibility of the attending midwife

- Where there is any doubt about when the fetus or fetuses have died, register as a stillbirth

FOLLOW-UP

- Give parents adequate time to discuss issues and ask questions before discharge. They may wish to speak to the midwife looking after them, obstetric staff or specialist midwife for bereavement services

- Give parents information and support contact numbers before discharge

- Arrange follow-up appointment with named obstetric consultant. In some circumstances and with the agreement of all parties, it may be more appropriate to arrange an appointment with the consultant who has been involved in mother's care while in hospital

In the community

- After discharge, the majority of parents who have lost a baby will require care and support in the community

- Specialist midwife for bereavement services may (in conjunction with community midwife/GP where appropriate) visit parents at home

- GP and community midwife will be informed of delivery. When delivery has occurred <24 weeks, woman may choose not to have a community midwife visit; >24 weeks, there is a statutory requirement for community midwife to visit

Issue 3
Issued: April 2015
Expires: April 2017

INTRODUCTION

Read this guideline in conjunction with the Caesarean section guideline

Risk of failed intubation in the obstetric population is approximately 10 times greater than in non-obstetric population. As this is associated with maternal morbidity and mortality it is strongly recommended that general anaesthesia (GA) is to be avoided if possible

PRE-OPERATIVE ASSESSMENT

The incidence of failed intubation with obesity has a 6% increase in odds with every 1 kg/m² increase in BMI

- Perform an anaesthetic risk assessment at antenatal clinic through an anaesthetic referral to:
- provide counselling for woman
- prepare a team management plan

Risk factors for identifying difficult intubation

- Previous surgery, radiotherapy or injury to head and neck
- History of difficult intubation
- Congenital craniofacial abnormalities
- Raised BMI at booking and full term
- Large protruding incisors
- Restricted neck movement (full, unhindered range of at least 90º)
- Restricted mouth opening (>3 fingers breadth), jaw slide
- Abnormal mallampati view (pharynx should be visible)

Consent

- Obtain and record consent
- Discuss:
- rapid sequence induction
- awake extubation
- increased recovery period
- failed intubation

Antacid regimen

- **High-risk labouring women** – ranitidine 150 mg oral 6-hrly
- **Elective lower segment caesarean section (LSCS)** – ranitidine 150 mg night before and on morning of surgery
- **Emergency LSCS** – ranitidine 50 mg IV (if not already receiving orally)
- **Sodium citrate:** 30 mL of 0.3 M sodium citrate drink within 20 min of anaesthesia for all grade 1–3 GA caesarean section and, if local policy, grade 4 caesarean section

PRE-INTUBATION PREPARATION

If difficult intubation envisaged, call for senior help

Equipment

- Appropriately checked anaesthetic machine
- Oro-pharyngeal airways and laryngeal masks
- Range of endotracheal tubes (ETT)
- Gum elastic bougie
- Range of laryngoscopes
- Airtraq optical laryngoscope, (only to be used by those with prior experience)
- Other difficult airway adjuncts as per local protocol (McCoy blades/ short handled laryngoscope/ video-laryngoscopes/ILMA/Proseal LMA/Aintree catheter)
- Cricothyrotomy kits

INTUBATION

- Confirm sodium citrate and ranitidine have been given, if not, consider IV ranitidine 50 mg slowly after induction
- Establish free-running IV infusion with a 16 G (or larger) cannula
- Position woman supine on table with a 15º left lateral tilt
- Give appropriate antibiotics – according to local practice

Pre-oxygenation

- Pre-oxygenate for 3 min with 100% oxygen via a close-fitting face mask, ensuring sufficient flow to prevent re-breathing
- Use high-flow oxygen (10 L/min) to improve speed of oxygenation of lungs

Monitoring

- Establish full monitoring as per Association of Anaesthetists of Great Britain and Ireland (AAGBI) guidelines

Preparation

- Position head in optimal intubating position
- If obese woman, use ramped up position
- When surgeon ready, instruct anaesthetic assistant to apply cricoid pressure

Anaesthetic administration

- Ensure good IV flow and administer a rapid bolus dose of at least 5 mg/kg thiopentone
- follow with suxamethonium 1 mg/kg
- in high risk woman, consider use of short-acting opiate to obtund sympathetic response
- Intubate when fasciculation ceased and woman relaxed
- Inflate cuff
- check no audible leak around cuff
- confirm correct placement with auscultation and capnography
- release cricoid pressure
- Once suxamethonium has worn off, give atracurium or rocuronium
- Maintain anaesthesia with oxygen and air or oxygen and nitrous oxide (usually 50% N_2O pre-delivery and 67% post-delivery), with an inhalational agent (isoflurane/sevoflurane) to keep a MAC of at least one
- Remember the possibility of patient awareness at all times

Intubation hints

- **If in doubt, take it out**
- A smaller ETT may be required in the presence of respiratory tract infection (URTI) or pre-eclamptic toxaemia (PET)
- Careful readjustment of applied cricoid pressure can improve view of the larynx
- Consider using a McCoy laryngoscope
- Use a short handled laryngoscope to overcome obstruction caused by woman's breasts
- If resistance faced, use a gum-elastic bougie for an anterior larynx. Rotate 90° anti-clockwise
- If resistance still present, release cricoid pressure

> *Remember – patients do not die from failure to intubate. They can die from prolonged attempts to intubate in the face of hypoxia and from unrecognised oesophageal intubation*

AFTER DELIVERY

- After cord clamped, give opioid (e.g. fentanyl 100 microgram and morphine 10 mg. Alternatively, if epidural *in situ*, top up with local anaesthetic and epidural opioid
- At end of surgery, and if not contraindicated, give 100 mg diclofenac rectally
- Perform TAP blocks at the end of surgery for post-operative pain relief
- Extubate woman awake in left lateral position in theatre
- Obese women may benefit from waking up in the upright position

Transfer to recovery room

- Transfer to recovery room for a minimum of 30 min
- See **Recovery** guideline

Issue 3
Issued: April 2015
Expires: April 2017

FAILED INTUBATION

If laryngoscopy or intubation is deemed impossible, institute failed intubation procedure without delay

- **Call for consultant anaesthetist help urgently**
- Consider simple changes in technique (head position, laryngoscope blade, alteration of cricoid pressure)

Do not waste time on repeated attempts at intubation, it can turn 'cannot intubate' to 'cannot ventilate airway'

Repeated attempts at intubation are associated with increased airway and haemodynamic complications

- Do not give second dose of suxamethonium
- Consider use of oropharyngeal airway, LMA or Proseal LMA if ventilation impossible. Release cricoid pressure to place LMA
- If it does not compromise ventilation, maintain cricoid pressure once LMA in place
- Do not turn woman onto her side
- Ventilate with 100% oxygen with bag and mask
- If ventilation still impossible, perform cricothyroidotomy
- Wake woman and consider alternatives (spinal, awake intubation)

Decision NOT to wake mother

- Will depend on the following factors:
- Woman's life at risk:
- cardiac arrest
- massive haemorrhage
- Baby's life at risk:
- severe fetal distress

Infiltration anaesthesia

- May be considered in severe fetal distress if mother consents and staff are familiar with this technique

Despite adequate ventilation, if you believe woman's life to be at risk, without a protected/definite airway, wake her until senior help arrives

Anaesthesia with spontaneous respiration

- Deepen anaesthesia with Sevoflurane (non-irritant)
- **Do not** manipulate airway in order to promote airway compromise or induce vomiting
- **Do not** attempt intubation through an LMA or fibre optic intubation under these circumstances, as this may result in an obstructed airway, oesophageal intubations, regurgitation, cardiac arrest
- **Remember**, cricothrotomy has poor results in inexperienced hands

Extubation strategy

- Ensure senior help has arrived
- Evaluate general clinical factors that may have an adverse impact on ventilation before extubation
- Consider a strategy for reintubation if necessary
- Always perform an awake extubation

Follow-up care

- Document description of airway difficulties encountered (in ventilation and intubation). Include airway management techniques employed
- Council woman appropriately post-operatively
- Follow-up for potential complications: oedema, bleeding, tracheal and esophageal perforation, pneumothorax and aspiration

Failed intubation during rapid sequence induction (RSI) in an obstetric patient

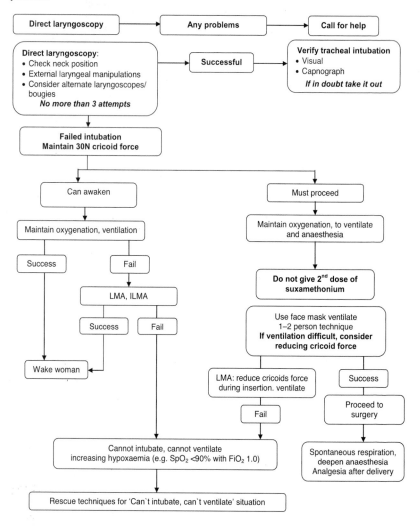

Issue 3
Issued: April 2015
Expires: April 2017

Neonatal herpes is a rare (1.7/10,000 in the UK) but serious disease with a significant mortality

Causes

May be caused by herpes simplex virus type 1 (HSV-1) or herpes simplex virus type 2 (HSV-2)

Transmission

Transmission of virus from mother to fetus occurs mostly by direct contact with virus in the genital tract during birth, although cases of transplacental infection and postnatal transmission have been reported

Maternal infection

May be primary or recurrent

Primary infection

- Risks are greatest in the third trimester, particularly within six weeks of delivery, as viral shedding may persist and baby is likely to be born before the development of protective maternal antibodies

Recurrent infection

- Is associated with a very low risk of neonatal herpes
- Recurrent herpes at the time of delivery causes localised forms of neonatal herpes only

ANTENATAL DIAGNOSIS AND MANAGEMENT

- Refer women who present with lesions that are thought to be herpes to genitourinary medicine (GUM). Make it clear the woman is pregnant
- GUM clinic will arrange screening for other sexually transmitted infections
- Active herpes is painful and analgesia may be required
- Ask directly whether woman can pass urine. It is not unusual for an indwelling catheter to be required

Antiretroviral therapy

- Women with a history of recurrent herpes may reduce the risk of active lesions at time of delivery by taking oral aciclovir for the last four weeks of pregnancy. Refer them to GUM for further discussion
- If woman develops primary infection before or earlier in pregnancy, prophylactic oral aciclovir is not recommended in the last four weeks of pregnancy

DELIVERY

Mode of delivery

- If woman develops her first episode of active herpes after 28 weeks' gestation or within six weeks of the onset of labour, offer delivery by caesarean section
- There is no indication to deliver a woman by caesarean section because of a history of genital herpes before pregnancy or earlier in pregnancy
- Advise women with active recurrent herpes lesions at the onset of labour that the risk of neonatal herpes is very small and that caesarean section is not routinely recommended

Care in labour

Primary infection

- If woman refuses delivery by caesarean section, avoid fetal scalp electrodes, fetal blood sampling and, where possible, instrumental delivery to minimise risk of vertical transmission
- Inform neonatologists during labour
- Give aciclovir, 5 mg/kg (350 mg for a 70 kg woman) IV 8-hrly over 60 min

Recurrent infection

- Women with active recurrent genital herpes and confirmed rupture of membranes – augment labour as soon as possible
- In women with active recurrent genital herpes, avoid invasive procedures during labour and inform neonatologists

BACKGROUND

- Group B streptococcus (GBS) disease in the newborn is defined as **early onset** within first 7 days of life – over 90% present within first 24 hr of birth
- often with rapid onset in first hours after birth
- There is a 10% mortality rate in affected neonates
- Risk can be reduced by giving maternal intrapartum antibiotics – see **Intrapartum antibiotics** below
- Late onset cannot be prevented

ANTENATAL MANAGEMENT

- Routine antenatal screening not recommended

GBS detected in current pregnancy

MSSU positive

- Recommend antenatal and intrapartum antibiotics
- **Antenatal antibiotics** – oral penicillin preparations. If allergic to penicillin, according to sensitivities (e.g. erythromycin) and local guidance. If none available, discuss with microbiologist
- **Intrapartum antibiotics** – see **Intrapartum antibiotics** below
- Clearly document the need for intrapartum antibiotics in maternal healthcare record

Vaginal swab positive

From high vaginal swab (HVS)/ low vaginal swab (LVS)

- If detected at any gestation, advise delivery on consultant-led unit and advise intrapartum antibiotic prophylaxis (IAP) – see **Intrapartum antibiotics** below
- Antenatal antibiotics are **not** recommended as GBS is normal vaginal flora for many women
- Clearly document the need for intrapartum antibiotics in maternal healthcare record

INTRAPARTUM MANAGEMENT

Indications for intrapartum antibiotics

- Any one of the following:
- previous infant with invasive GBS disease; arrange consultant-led unit care
- GBS bacteriuria this pregnancy
- GBS on vaginal swab in this pregnancy
- fever ≥38°C during labour at any gestation
- Inform mother of the risk of adverse reaction to antibiotics and that, despite attempts at prophylaxis, some babies will still acquire infection
- In women with GBS and spontaneous rupture of membranes at term in the absence of labour, advise immediate induction of labour with intrapartum antibiotics once in labour

Intrapartum antibiotics

- Vaginal delivery – give **mother** benzylpenicillin 3 g IV in 100 mL sodium chloride 0.9% over 10 min then 1.5 g 4-hrly until delivery
- if allergic to penicillin, give clindamycin 900 mg IV in 50 mL sodium chloride 0.9% over 30 min 8-hrly until delivery
- give intrapartum antibiotics as soon as possible after the onset of labour and at least 2 hr before delivery

Antibiotic prophylaxis not indicated

- Caesarean section – no investigation or treatment necessary if intact membrane, no suspicion of chorioamnionitis and no maternal fever

> *If chorioamnionitis suspected, give broad-spectrum antibiotics, which will also cover Group B streptococcal disease*

NEONATE

Risk factors for infection

- Maternity service to inform neonatal service of risk factors:
- pre-labour rupture of membranes
- preterm birth (<37 weeks), especially with pre-labour rupture of membranes
- confirmed or suspected chorioamnioitis (e.g. intrapartum fever)
- invasive group B streptococcal (GBS) infection in a previous baby
- antibiotic treatment given to mother for confirmed or suspected invasive bacterial infection 24 hr before, during, or post labour
- Breastfeeding does not increase risk of neonatal GBS disease

Observations

- If antibiotics indicated but not given or received an inadequate dose of IAP, observe baby for 12–24 hr after birth on postnatal ward with regular assessment of:
- general wellbeing
- feeding
- heart rate
- respiratory rate
- temperature

Recognition and assessment

- Signs of early GBS infection are non specific and could include:
- grunting/tachypnoea/respiratory distress
- pallor/cyanosis
- lethargy
- irritability
- poor feeding
- tachycardia/bradycardia
- hypotension
- Treat all babies from a multiple pregnancy if infection suspected in one
- For red flag signs, risk factors, and clinical indicators for treatment, follow **Infection in first 72 hours of life** guideline in the Staffordshire, Shropshire & Black Country Newborn and Maternity Network Neonatal guidelines

HEPATITIS B

Introduction

Hepatitis B is a blood borne viral infection affecting the liver. It is caused by the Hepatitis B virus (HBV) transferred in blood or body fluid

Principles of isolation

- Body fluids are regarded as infectious material. Take appropriate infection control precautions in line with local Trust policy

Antenatal care

- As part of antenatal care, provide all women with information on, and access to, HBV screening
- If mother positive for HBV:
- review in consultant-led antenatal clinic, where an individualised management plan will be drawn up
- alert neonatal team and inform public health team and GP of plan to immunise
- Arrange for prophylaxis according to local guidance
- Refer women with HBV infection to a consultant with expertise in liver disease for further assessment

Intrapartum care

- When an HBsAg positive mother arrives in labour or for caesarean section, inform on-call neonatal team
- **Avoid fetal scalp sampling and fetal scalp electrodes**
- Hepatitis B infection is not an indication for caesarean section as there is insufficient evidence that it reduces mother-to-child transmission
- If woman requires in-utero transfer, immunoglobulin (if indicated) must accompany her
- If unbooked or untested woman accepts testing, send sample for antenatal screening to microbiology urgently (notify microbiologist on duty/on-call via switchboard) to allow immunisation within 24 hr of delivery if required

Postnatal care

- For all newborns, check antenatal screening results for mother's tests
- If antenatal testing not done (e.g. concealed pregnancy) request urgent maternal hepatitis B virus surface antigen (HBsAg) test and other infection screening bloods (HIV and syphilis) – see **HIV positive women** guideline
- Wash baby immediately following birth and cleanse the oropharynx and nasal cavities of all visible maternal blood and secretions by gentle wiping
- Encourage and support breastfeeding (unless mother also HIV+) but do not allow mother to donate milk as the virus has been detected in breast milk
- Inform postnatal ward baby will require immunisation

Communication

- Give mother information about Hepatitis B, modes of transmission and prevention of spread
- Obtain parental consent for immunisation

IMMEDIATE POSTNATAL TREATMENT OF BABY

Immunisation

- Some babies require Hepatitis B immunoglobulin (HBIG) as well as immunisation
- Order immunoglobulin [HBIG antenatally if required (see **Table**)], depending on mother's antigen status
- Immunise baby of HBsAg positive mother as follows, depending on other hepatitis B markers in mother during pregnancy:

Issue 3
Issued: April 2015
Expires: April 2017

Maternal status	Vaccine required by baby	Immunoglobulin (HBIG) required by baby
HBsAg positive, HBeAg positive	Y	Y
HBsAg positive, HBeAg negative, HBe antibody (anti-HBe) negative	Y	Y
HBsAg positive where e markers have not been determined	Y	Y
Acute hepatitis B during pregnancy	Y	Y
HBsAg positive and baby <1.5 kg	Y	Y
HBsAg positive, anti-HBe positive	Y	N
HBsAg positive and >106 iu/mL Hepatitis B DNA in antenatal sample	Y	Y
Other high risk group (e.g. HIV)	Y	N

● Give low-birth-weight and premature babies full neonatal dose of hepatitis B vaccine

● Give HBIG and hepatitis B vaccine to babies with birth weight <1.5 kg born to mother with hepatitis B, regardless of mother's HBeAg status

● obtain HBIG from regional virus laboratory service or local microbiology as applicable

● Give hepatitis B vaccine to HIV exposed/infected neonates

When

● Give first immunisation +/– HBIG within 24 hr of delivery on postnatal ward. Check that arrangements are in place for further immunisations and follow-up to be provided in the community or by paediatrician – see **Hepatitis B and C** guideline in the Staffordshire, Shropshire & Black Country Newborn and Maternity Network Neonatal guidelines (if used locally)

What

● Hepatitis B vaccine, 0.5 mL IM. Caution: brands have different doses [e.g. engerix-B® 10 microgram (recommended), HBVaxPro Paediatric® 5 microgram]

● HBIG 200 units additionally IM in opposite thigh to that of the Hepatitis B vaccine soon after birth and no later than 24 hr simultaneously with vaccine to babies of highly infectious mothers (see **Table** above)

● Three further doses of hepatitis B vaccine will be given according to local policy at one month, two months and one year of age

How

● Use two separate injection sites for hepatitis B vaccine and HBIG, in anterolateral aspect of the thighs (not buttocks)

● Give hepatitis B vaccine IM, except in bleeding disorder where it may be given deep subcutaneously

Dose regimen for infants of mothers with Hepatitis B

● Vaccine is given at 0, 1, 2 and 12 months

● Book hospital out-patient appointment for 12 months for testing for HBsAg

● see the Staffordshire, Shropshire & Black Country Newborn and Maternity Network Neonatal **Hepatitis B and C** guideline (if used locally)

Relationship to other immunisations

- No need to delay BCG following HBIG
- Hepatitis B vaccine may be given with other vaccines, but use separate site. If same limb used, give vaccines >2.5 cm apart

HEPATITIS IMMUNISATION

To whom

- Hepatitis B immunisation is recommended with other routine immunisations for high risk babies born to mothers:
- with partners who are hepatitis B surface antigen (HBsAg) positive
- who are or with partners who are IV drug users (even if HBsAg negative)
- who change sexual partners frequently (e.g. commercial sex workers)
- with close family contacts known to be HBsAg positive
- who intend to live in a country with high prevalence of hepatitis B (Africa, Asia, Eastern Europe, Northern Canada, Alaska)

Dose regimen for infants of mothers HBsAg negative with other indications for vaccination

- Vaccine is given at 0, 1 and 6 months – see **Hepatitis B and C** guideline in the Staffordshire, Shropshire & Black Country Newborn and Maternity Network Neonatal guidelines (if used locally)

HEPATITIS C

Introduction

- Hepatitis C is a blood borne viral infection carrying a high risk of chronic infection and liver disease. Only 1–2% of pregnant women are anti HCV positive in the UK
- It is caused by the Hepatitis C virus (HCV) transferred in blood and body fluids

High risk groups

- Current or former intravenous drug use or women with partners who are IV drug users
- From a country of high prevalence [e.g. North Africa (particularly Egypt), Middle East]

Principles of isolation

- All body fluids are considered infectious material. Take appropriate infection control precautions in line with local Trust policy

Antenatal care

- A test for HCV infection is not part of routine antenatal screening, but should be offered to women who report a history of IV drug use in themselves or their partner, and to women who believe they had a positive test for HCV Ab in the past. A positive HCV RNA report confirms current HCV infection
- Refer pregnant women with HCV infection to a consultant with expertise in liver disease for further assessment
- Reassure woman with HCV infection that pregnancy will not affect the course of the HCV infection and HCV infection will not affect the course of the pregnancy, and that the risk of mother-to-child transmission of HCV is low in the absence of HIV infection
- Alert neonatal team

Intrapartum care

- **Avoid fetal scalp blood sampling and fetal scalp electrodes**
- Because of increased risk of fetal abrasion or scalp trauma, avoid difficult instrumental delivery
- Hepatitis C infection is not an indication for caesarean section, as there is insufficient evidence that it reduces mother-to-child transmission. However, if woman is co-infected with HIV, caesarean section is indicated

Issue 3
Issued: April 2015
Expires: April 2017

Postnatal care

- Presence of passively acquired maternal antibodies that can persist in infants until 15–18 months of age renders anti-HCV Ab detection of limited value for diagnosis of infection. To investigate vertical transmission, review child at 18 months and 3 and 12 years

- There is no contraindication to breastfeeding unless dual HCV and HIV infection – see **HIV positive women** guideline

INTRODUCTION

- High dependency care on delivery suite provides an intermediate level of care between that on a ward and Intensive Care Unit (ICU). This can be level 1 and 2 critical care
- Women requiring multiple organ support or requiring mechanical ventilation (level 3 care) will require transfer to an ICU

PRINCIPLES OF MANAGEMENT

- To care for women who have been recognised as unwell using the MEWS system to safely provide more frequent observation and monitoring in individual clinical cases
- To provide individualised multidisciplinary care
- To stabilise woman before transfer to critical care facilities

EQUIPMENT

- Ensure stock levels of appropriate equipment in the room used are maintained and checked as per local practice
- Resuscitation trolley with defibrillator and airway management equipment
- Resuscitation/emergency drugs
- Monitoring equipment and accessories for:
- pulse
- BP
- ECG
- SaO_2 and with transducer facility for invasive monitoring
- Equipment for insertion and management of invasive monitoring (arterial and CVP)
- Piped oxygen and suction
- Intravenous fluid warmer
- Forced air warming device
- Infusion pumps

Available on delivery suite/unit

- Blood gas analyser
- Emergency massive haemorrhage equipment
- Emergency eclampsia equipment
- O-ve blood
- Intravenous fluid warmers, forced air warming devices
- Transfer equipment – monitor and ventilator

Issue 3
Issued: April 2015
Expires: April 2017

LEVELS OF CRITICAL CARE

Level 0	Needs can be met through normal ward care
Level 1	Women at risk of deterioration and requiring a higher level of observation
Level 2	Invasive monitoring/intervention required that includes support for a single failing organ (excluding advanced respiratory support) **Basic respiratory support** ≥50% oxygen via face mask to maintain oxygen saturation **Basic cardiovascular support** ● IV anti-hypertensives e.g. pre-eclampsia ● CVP and arterial line management **Advanced cardiovascular support** ● Simultaneous use of at least 2 anti-arrhythmic/anti-hypertensive/vasoactive drugs IV **Neurological support** ● Magnesium infusion to control seizures ● Hepatic support Management of HELLP syndrome or acute fatty liver
Level 3	Advanced respiratory support required (mechanical ventilation) alone or basic respiratory support together with support of at least one additional organ **Advanced respiratory support** ● Invasive mechanical ventilation **Support of two or more organ systems**

INDICATIONS FOR LEVEL 1 AND 2 CRITICAL CARE

- This list is not exhaustive
- Women requiring invasive monitoring
- Modified early warning score (MEWS) >6, or an increasing score despite intervention
- Women requiring invasive monitoring
- Severe pregnancy-induced hypertension
- PET, eclampsia, HELLP syndrome
- Obstetric haemorrhage >1.5 L
- causing maternal CVS compromise
- requiring acute transfusion >4 units blood
- Severe infection/sepsis
- Sudden unexplained collapse
- Disseminated intravascular coagulation (DIC)
- Diabetic ketoacidosis
- Certain medical or surgical conditions compromising maternal condition

Staff responsibilities

- Women requiring maternal critical care must be discussed with the senior obstetrician and co-ordinating midwife
- Midwives caring for the woman should be trained to do so or under the supervision of a critical care trained midwife (see below)
- If woman receiving critical care, level 1 or greater, provide one-to-one care

- Clinical decisions should be made jointly by obstetricians, anaesthetists and midwives
- In women with significant system compromise, involve senior clinicians from other disciplines early
- Consultant obstetric anaesthetist and consultant obstetrician should review all women receiving level 2 care at least twice daily, and women receiving level 1 care at least once a day
- Inform obstetric and anaesthetic consultants early of any changes in clinical condition
- There should be a detailed handover between clinicians at the end of each shift

ON COMMENCEMENT OF HIGH DEPENDENCY CARE

- A management plan formulated to include as a minimum: - fluid balance, frequency of observations and type of monitoring required, thromboprophylaxis risk assessment and analgesia
- Clearly document handover to and from maternal critical care
- Provide and document the following information given to woman and her family:
- reason for high dependency care
- explanation of procedures, drugs and care given

MONITORING

Observations

- Undertake observations at frequency according to guidance for the underlying diagnosis and document in appropriate charts:
- temperature
- pulse
- respiratory rate
- oxygen saturations
- blood pressure
- fluid balance

CONSIDERATIONS FOR TRANSFER TO CRITICAL CARE AREA

- When woman requires:
- level 3 critical care or respiratory support
- level 2 critical care which cannot be provided on delivery suite
- level 2 critical care of >1 organ/system
- level 2 critical care currently but at a significant risk of deterioration
- Start intensive care when it is needed with early involvement of ICU consultant. Do not delay until admission to ICU

> *Decision to transfer woman to critical care area must be made by consultant obstetrician and consultant anaesthetist after discussion with intensive care specialists*

Transfer

- Ensure documentation from all staff groups is complete as per local guidance, with details of how to contact them if further information is required
- Complete relevant transfer documentation including handover tool
- Refer to **Maternal transfer** guideline

Discharge to non-maternity wards

- Where maternal condition dictates that ongoing care is required by another speciality, identify a named non-obstetric consultant to liaise with named obstetrician
- Named obstetrician is responsible for ensuring regular obstetric reviews
- Woman to be formally handed over at each change of staff on labour ward
- If woman is discharged home from a non-obstetric ward, labour ward co-ordinator must be informed to ensure community midwife is notified of discharge

DISCHARGE FROM HDU

- Decision to discharge is made in consultation between obstetrician, anaesthetist and midwife, provided:
- all observations are stable and organ support no longer required
- woman is alert and orientated and no longer requires observation or treatment available on HDU
- obstetrician has written an on-going plan of care
- there has been careful handover to the receiving ward using local handover tool
- After leaving HDU care, senior medical staff must review woman
- Provide woman with information about what has happened and encourage her to participate in decisions relating to recovery

Check latest version of individualised maternal care plan

TESTING

- Recommend HIV testing to all pregnant women as a routine part of antenatal screening

- if HIV testing declined, offer counselling by HIV specialist (if available)

- Check HIV test result in notes at every visit: if no result available, recommend retesting. If not done early in pregnancy, offer at 28 weeks' gestation

- If in labour and no HIV test result, request urgent testing with consent

ANTENATAL CARE

- Ensure consultant-led antenatal care in conjunction with HIV physician and, if available, HIV specialist nurses

- Advise mother not to breastfeed and ensure she has formula and steriliser

- Ensure stock of IV zidovudine and oral suspensions zidovudine, lamivudine and nevirapine on labour ward

- See woman's individualised HIV care plan

During pregnancy

- Amniocentesis or chorionic villus sampling should only be performed with antiviral cover

- If a woman taking antiretrovirals presents with GI upset, fatigue, fever and breathlessness, check lactate levels: if raised do not give antiretrovirals and inform HIV team

MODE OF DELIVERY

- Women known to be HIV positive will have been counselled antenatally and a plan made for mode of delivery and care on delivery suite

- Normal vaginal delivery is now recommended for women:

- with a viral load of <50 copies/mL who have been treated antenatally with highly active antiviral therapy (HAART)

- who are elite controllers (have a viral load of <50 copies/mL untreated) and who have been on zidovudine monotherapy (IV zidovudine in labour is not required)

- For women with a viral load of 50–400 copies/mL who have been treated antenatally with HAART, consider pre-labour caesarean section (CS), taking into account:

- actual viral load

- trajectory of viral load

- length of time on treatment

- adherence issues

- obstetric factors

- woman's views

- Pre-labour CS is advised for women with:

- a viral load of >50 copies/mL who were not taking HAART, including women on zidovudine monotherapy

- a viral load of >400 copies/mL for those who were taking HAART

- Arrange pre-labour CS at 38–39 weeks' gestation

INTRAPARTUM INTRAVENOUS ZIDOVUDINE

Indications

- Women with a viral load >1,000 copies/mL

- Untreated women with an unknown viral load

- Women on zidovudine monotherapy. An alternative for these women is to continue their oral regime

- There is no evidence that intrapartum IV zidovudine is beneficial for women taking HAART with a viral load of <1,000 copies/mL

Issue 3
Issued: April 2015
Expires: April 2017

Medication

- Start zidovudine IV 4 hr before elective CS (or for as long as possible before emergency CS):
- prepare an infusion of 2 mg/mL in glucose 5%
- run 1 mL/kg/hr for first hour (for a 70 kg woman this is 70 mL/hr)
- after one hour, reduce rate to 0.5 mL/kg/hr (for a 70 kg woman this is 35 mL/hr)
- use actual body weight even if >100 kg
- Stop infusion after cord is clamped

VAGINAL DELIVERY

- Manage women with careful infection control procedures
- In women for whom intrapartum IV zidovudine is indicated, see **Medication** above. It may be necessary to contact on-call pharmacist to ensure adequate supply of zidovudine
- If pre-labour rupture of membranes occurs at term, or in any gestation after 34 weeks, commence oxytocin without delay – see **Oxytocin** guideline
- If labour is progressing normally, avoid amniotomy
- Be vigilant for pyrexia in labour and have low threshold for antibiotic therapy
- Continue oral HAART medication throughout labour
- Fetal blood sampling and fetal scalp electrodes are not contraindicated for woman with viral load <50 copies/mL taking HAART
- If instrumental delivery required, prefer low cavity forceps to Ventouse

PRETERM DELIVERY

<34 weeks' gestation

- In threatened preterm labour or if baby has absent/reversed end diastolic flow, if mother's viral load >50 copies/mL, administer nevirapine 200 mg oral once to mother to load baby who will be **unable to take oral medication after birth**

- give nevirapine >2 hr before birth if possible
- Discuss with HIV consultant the use of double dose tenofovir +/- raltegravir to reduce risk of vertical transmission
- Continue mother's current antiviral therapy
- If preterm pre-labour rupture of membranes occurs, on-call consultant obstetrician will weigh the risk of prematurity and vertical transmission. Most recent viral load can be helpful
- There is no contraindication to steroids for mother to reduce risk of RDS in baby

TERM RUPTURE OF MEMBRANES

- In all cases of term pre-labour spontaneous rupture of the membranes, expedite delivery following woman's individual HIV care plan for birth
- If indicated in individual care plan, prepare for caesarean section as soon as the zidovudine infusion is commenced at initial rate. Do not wait to complete before delivering baby

CAESAREAN SECTION

Preparation

- Midwife co-ordinator informs theatre team of woman's HIV status, which **must not** be recorded on theatre list
- For women who require intrapartum IV zidovudine
- because delivery must occur during the zidovudine infusion, ensure first or very early on theatre list
- If first on list, admit the night before for IV cannula before midnight. Woman must take oral antiretrovirals at usual times before caesarean section (CS) even if nil-by-mouth
- Antibiotic prophylaxis is particularly important due to increased risk of postpartum fever

Precautions

- All healthcare professionals performing or assisting at a CS where woman is known to be HIV positive should wear double gloves to reduce risk of transmission

AFTER DELIVERY

- **High risk** (maternal viral load >50 or unknown): give baby zidovudine, lamivudine and nevirapine <2 hr from birth

- **Low-risk** (maternal viral load <50 in last 4 weeks): give baby zidovudine <4 hr of delivery

- Contact neonatal team while mother still on delivery suite

- Follow mother's individualised HIV care plan with regard to discontinuing antivirals

- Prescribe cabergoline 1 mg single dose first day postpartum to all mothers to inhibit lactation. Maternal hypertension is a contraindication

- Take 5 mL EDTA sample from mother to go with baby's sample for HIV DNA PCR testing

- For neonatal care see Staffordshire, Shropshire & Black Country Newborn and Maternity Network **Neonatal HIV** guideline (if used locally)

- Ensure woman has follow-up with her HIV physician and team in two weeks

COMMUNICATION WITH WOMAN

- Inform woman that:
- giving birth is generally very safe for both her and her baby
- there is a higher likelihood of a normal birth with less intervention among women who plan to give birth at home
- there are rare events that, if occurring at home, may have worse outcome for mother and baby than if occurring in hospital

> *Midwives undertaking home births must be competent in obstetric and neonatal emergencies and must attend annual mandatory update training*

Referral for home birth

- On confirmation of pregnancy, woman can either refer herself to a community midwife who is attached to a GP surgery, or ask GP to refer her

MANAGEMENT PLAN

Community midwife

- Takes a comprehensive booking history and performs risk assessment
- Offers woman choice of planning a birth at home, in a midwife-led unit or in an obstetric-led unit (NICE 2007 CG 55 Intrapartum care), according to assessed risk
- Provides antenatal care
- Provides contact details, together with those of the local maternity unit and documents in maternal healthcare record
- Arranges booking scan. Subsequent mid-trimester scan will be arranged at initial booking scan visit
- Encourages woman to attend regular antenatal visits as per local care pathways

- Completes notification of home birth as per local policy
- While home birth is predominantly a choice available for women meeting the low-risk criteria, occasionally women who **do not** fit this criteria may request a home birth. In these cases, see **High-risk care** overleaf
- **34–36 weeks' gestation:**
- carries out risk assessment and discusses home birth arrangements/ birth plan
- **36–37 weeks' gestation:**
- checks and arranges delivery of home birth equipment to woman's home
- Women **must be** informed of possible complications during labour and delivery which may necessitate transfer to hospital via ambulance
- midwife must document in detail that discussion has taken place

> *If, at any time, woman's risk category changes, appropriate referral must be made*

Pethidine

- Follow local policy for making pethidine available
- Midwife checks and administers the injection of pethidine according to NMC standards for medicines management (2008) and NMC Rules and Standards (2004)

Home birth cover

- Woman contacts the maternity hospital as discussed during her birth plan visit
- The maternity unit will contact a midwife as per local arrangements
- Community midwife will ensure all equipment is available and attend woman
- refer to local **Lone worker** policy
- Once labour diagnosed, second midwife will be requested

Intrapartum care at home birth

- First midwife is responsible/accountable for care in labour and delivery
- Second midwife attends and supports first midwife during delivery and with any obstetric/neonatal emergency as required
- Intrapartum care record is used to record progress of labour and delivery
- Intrapartum auscultation of the fetal heart using a sonic aid – see **Intermittent auscultation** guideline. If deviations from normal are identified at any time during home birth, midwives must act accordingly (NMC guidelines September 2007) see **Maternal transfer** guideline (or follow local practice) **and NMC midwives rules**
- Local maternity hospital must be informed when labour and placenta delivery are complete

Born before arrival

- If born at home, unattended by a midwife, follow local **Born before arrival** policy
- Consider safeguarding issues. Depending on condition of woman and/or baby, admission to hospital via paramedic ambulance may be necessary

POSTNATAL CARE AT A HOME BIRTH

Mother

- As routine, record:
- temperature
- pulse
- BP
- Suture if required see **Perineal trauma suturing (tears and episiotomy)** guideline
- Initiate skin-to-skin contact and breast or bottle feeding according to woman's preference and document time – see Staffordshire, Shropshire & Black Country Newborn and Maternity Network neonatal **Breastfeeding** guideline or follow local practice
- If breastfeeding, arrange breastfeeding support
- Assist mother with personal hygiene
- Provide local contact numbers and tell mother who to contact for emergency medical relief (e.g. 999)

Baby

- As routine following delivery:
- obtain parental consent and administer vitamin K (Konakion MM paediatric) 0.1 mL IM

General

First midwife

- Arranges home visit for next day or later that day if required (depending on time of delivery)
- Returns equipment to local maternity unit
- Obtains NHS number for baby
- Records delivery in maternal healthcare record
- Initiates Red book
- Restocks home birth bag as per local practice and records this has taken place
- Ensures neonatal resuscitation equipment is clean, complete and signed back in as per local practice
- Ensures entonox tubing is re-usable, Entonox cylinders **must** be replaced by contacting hospital porters
- On-call community midwives inform local maternity unit that they have returned home
- Arrange hearing screening for baby using appropriate request form
- Inform woman's GP that home delivery has taken place

HIGH-RISK CARE

- Women who are booked for high-risk care may also wish to deliver their baby at home, and have a right to do so

- Midwives discuss woman's wishes with her in a non-judgemental manner, providing detailed information, options for care and outlining any potential risks so that the woman may make a fully informed decision about place of delivery

- If in line with local policy, offer high-risk woman the opportunity to deliver on the midwifery-led unit as a safer option, in agreement with her consultant, named midwife and unit manager

- A supervisor of midwives must be available (contact via delivery suite) at all times for advice

> *Good preparation is key.*
> *Midwives must not practice outside the scope of their abilities (NMC rules). He/she must ensure a supervisor of midwives is contacted and must not be drawn into unsafe practice*

- Consultant providing care will discuss woman's wishes with her

- Community midwife must make every effort to attend the appointment to ensure all parties have explored the risks of home birth. If it is not possible for the community midwife to attend the appointment, she should discuss with consultant before appointment date

- If a woman chooses not to accept the advice provided by the consultant and community midwife, make an appointment for her to meet with a supervisor of midwives to ensure all possibilities have been explained

Documentation

- Document all discussions between mother/community midwife/consultant/ supervisor of midwives in the maternal healthcare record

- Formulate a detailed plan (agreed by all parties) and place copies in:

- woman's hand held records

- local maternity unit

- woman's healthcare record

Hypertensive disorders during pregnancy occur in women with pre-existing primary or secondary chronic hypertension, and in women who develop new-onset hypertension in the second half of pregnancy (gestational hypertension)

> *If occurring with significant proteinuria it is termed pre-eclampsia – see Eclampsia and Severe pre-eclampsia guidelines*

DEFINITION

Chronic hypertension

● Hypertension present at booking visit or <20 weeks' gestation or if woman already taking antihypertensive medication when referred to maternity services. Can be primary or secondary in aetiology

Degrees of hypertension

Mild	Moderate	Severe
Systolic BP 140–149 mmHg	Systolic BP 150–159 mmHg	Systolic BP ≥160 mmHg
Diastolic BP 90–99 mmHg	Diastolic BP 100–109 mmHg	Diastolic BP ≥110 mmHg

RISKS

Woman

● Increase in lifetime risk of chronic hypertension and cardiovascular disease

Baby

● Higher rates of perinatal mortality, preterm and low birth weight

SYMPTOMS AND SIGNS

● Advise woman to report any of the following to a healthcare professional:

● headache

● visual disturbance (blurring or flashing)

● pain below ribs

● sudden swelling of face, hands or feet

● vomiting

INVESTIGATIONS

● BP and urinalysis on each visit to a healthcare professional

Gestational hypertension (GHT)

● New hypertension presenting after 20 weeks' gestation without significant proteinuria

GHT with significant proteinuria

● New hypertension presenting after 20 weeks' gestation with urinary protein: creatinine ratio >30 mg/mmol or a validated 24 hr urine collection result shows >300 mg protein

TREATMENT

Antihypertensive treatment and prenatal counselling

● Base antihypertensive treatment on pre-existing treatment, medication side-effect profile and risk of teratogenicity

● Stop angiotensin-converting enzyme inhibitors (ACEI) and/or angiotensin II receptor blockers (ARBs) **within 2 days** of notification of pregnancy and offer alternative medication

● ACEI and ARB carry an increased risk of congenital abnormalities

● Limited evidence shows no increased risk of congenital abnormalities with other antihypertensive treatments but discuss with healthcare professional responsible for managing the hypertension

● The antihypertensive medications commenced/used in pregnancy are methyldopa, labetalol and nifedipine

Issue 3
Issued: April 2015
Expires: April 2017

Postnatal care

Antihypertensive treatment

- Continue antenatal antihypertensive treatment
- If methyldopa was used during pregnancy, stop within 2 days of birth due to risk of depression
- If no antenatal antihypertensive treatment was required, commence antihypertensive treatment only if BP ≥150/100 mmHg
- Measure BP:
- daily for first 2 days after birth
- at least once 3–5 days after birth
- as clinically indicated if antihypertensive treatment changed
- Maintain BP at 140/90 mmHg
- See **Breastfeeding advice for women taking antihypertensive medication** below

Follow-up care

- At transfer to community care, ensure care plan in place, including:
- who will provide follow-up care (including medical review if required)
- frequency of blood pressure monitoring
- thresholds for reducing or stopping treatment
- indications for referral to primary care for blood pressure review
- If antihypertensive treatment is to be continued, offer medical review 2 weeks after transfer to community care
- Offer medical review at 6–8 week postnatal GP review
- If antihypertensive treatment is to be continued after the 6–8 week postnatal review, offer a specialist assessment of hypertension

Breastfeeding advice for women taking antihypertensive medication

- If breastfeeding or expressing milk, avoid diuretic treatment

- Inform woman the following antihypertensive drugs have no known adverse effects on babies receiving breast milk:
- labetalol
- nifedipine
- enalapril
- captopril
- atenolol
- metoprolol
- Inform woman that there is insufficient evidence regarding the safety of babies receiving breast milk where mother is receiving:
- angiotensin II receptor blockers (ARBs)
- amlodipine
- angiotensin-converting enzyme (ACE) inhibitors other than enalapril and captopril
- Assess clinical wellbeing of baby, especially adequacy of feeding, at least daily for first 2 days after delivery

CHRONIC HYPERTENSION

Antihypertensive treatment

- See **Antihypertensive treatment and prenatal counselling** above
- In uncomplicated chronic hypertension, maintain blood pressure at <150/100 mmHg
- In target-organ damage secondary to chronic hypertension (e.g., kidney disease), maintain BP at <140/90 mmHg
- Refer pregnant women with secondary chronic hypertension to a specialist in hypertensive disorders

Aspirin therapy

- 75 mg daily from 12 weeks until delivery

Antenatal care

- Consultant obstetrician as lead professional
- Plan additional antenatal consultations according to individual needs of woman and baby

Fetal monitoring

- At 28–30 and 32–34 weeks perform:
- ○ ultrasound for fetal growth and amniotic fluid volume assessment
- ○ umbilical artery Doppler velocimetry
- If results normal, do not repeat after 34 weeks unless clinically indicated
- If fetal activity abnormal, perform electronic fetal monitoring – see **Electronic fetal monitoring (EFM)** guideline

Timing of birth

- Chronic hypertension with blood pressure <160/110 mmHg, with or without antihypertensive treatment:
- ○ do not offer delivery before 37 weeks
- Chronic hypertension with blood pressure <160/110 mmHg after 37 weeks, with or without antihypertensive treatment:
- ○ after 37 weeks, woman and obstetrician will agree timing of birth
- Severe, uncontrolled chronic hypertension:
- ○ offer delivery after a course of corticosteroids completed (if required)

Intrapartum care

Mild or moderate hypertension (BP ≤159/109 mmHg)	Severe hypertension (BP ≥160/110 mmHg)
• Continue antenatal antihypertensive treatment • Measure BP hourly • See **Epidural analgesia** guideline – **Investigations** • If BP stable <150 mmHg systolic, do not routinely limit duration of second stage	• Continue antenatal antihypertensive treatment • Measure BP continuously • If BP controlled <150 mmHg systolic, do not routinely limit duration of second stage • If BP does not respond to initial treatment, advise operative birth

Postnatal care

See postnatal care above

GESTATIONAL HYPERTENSION WITHOUT PROTEINURIA

Prevention of GHT

Aspirin therapy

- Women with one or more high risk factors or two or more moderate risk factors of pre-eclampsia, start 75 mg aspirin daily from 12 weeks until delivery
- High risk factors:
- ○ hypertensive disease during a previous pregnancy
- ○ chronic kidney disease
- ○ autoimmune disease e.g. systemic lupus erythematosis or antiphospholipid syndrome

- ○ type 1 or type 2 diabetes
- ○ chronic hypertension
- Moderate risk factors:
- ○ first pregnancy
- ○ age ≥40 yr
- ○ pregnancy interval of >10 yr
- ○ body mass index (BMI) ≥35 kg/m^2 at first visit
- ○ family history of pre-eclampsia
- ○ multiple pregnancy

Antenatal care

- Assessment by middle grade obstetrician (ST3–7 or equivalent e.g. staff grade, clinical fellow) or consultant
- Consultant obstetrician as lead professional

Issue 3
Issued: April 2015
Expires: April 2017

Assessment and antihypertensive treatment (see **Antihypertensive treatment and prenatal counselling** above)

Mild hypertension (BP 140/90–149/99 mmHg)	Moderate hypertension (BP 150/100–159/109 mmHg)	Severe hypertension (BP ≥160/110 mmHg)
● Do not admit to hospital ● Do not treat hypertension ● Measure BP weekly ● Test for proteinuria at each visit using an automated reagent-strip reading device or urinary protein:creatinine ratio ● Perform routine antenatal blood tests ● If presenting at <32 weeks or at high risk of pre-eclampsia, test for proteinuria and measure BP twice a week	● Do not admit to hospital ● Treat with first-line oral labetalol to maintain BP at <150/80–100 mmHg (monitor via community midwife or assessment unit) ● Measure BP at least twice a week ● Test for proteinuria at each visit ● Test renal function, electrolytes, FBC, transaminases, bilirubin ● If no subsequent proteinuria, no further blood tests required	● Admit to hospital ● Keep mobile in hospital ● Treat with first-line oral labetalol to maintain BP at <150/80–100 mmHg ● Measure BP at least 4 times daily ● Test for proteinuria daily using an automated reagent-strip reading device or urinary protein:creatinine ratio ● Test LFT, U&E, FBC, transaminases, bilirubin at presentation and then monitor weekly ● If receiving out-patient care after severe hypertension has been effectively controlled in hospital: 　● measure BP and test for proteinuria twice a week 　● perform weekly blood tests

Fetal monitoring

Mild or moderate hypertension (BP 140/90–159/109 mmHg)	Severe hypertension (BP ≥160/110 mmHg)
● If diagnosis confirmed before 34 weeks, perform: 　● ultrasound for fetal growth and amniotic fluid volume assessment 　● umbilical artery Doppler velocimetry ● If results normal, do not repeat after 34 weeks ● If fetal activity abnormal: 　● EFM	● At diagnosis, if conservative management planned, perform: 　● ultrasound for fetal growth, amniotic fluid volume assessment and umbilical artery Doppler velocimetry (not >2-wkly) 　● EFM ● Do not repeat more than weekly if all fetal monitoring normal ● Repeat EFM if any of the following: 　● change in fetal movement reported by woman 　● vaginal bleeding 　● abdominal pain 　● deterioration in maternal condition ● If results of any fetal monitoring abnormal, inform consultant obstetrician

Timing of birth

- **GHT with blood pressure <160/110 mmHg,** with or without antihypertensive treatment
- do not offer delivery before 37 weeks
- **GHT with blood pressure <160/110 mmHg after 37 weeks,** with or without antihypertensive treatment
- woman and senior obstetrician agree timing of birth, and maternal and fetal indications for birth
- **Refractory severe gestational hypertension:**
- offer delivery after a course of corticosteroids (if required) has been completed

Intrapartum care for woman with GHT

Mild and moderate hypertension (BP 140/90–159/109 mmHg)	Severe hypertension (BP ≥160/110 mmHg)
<ul><li>BP hourly</li><li>Continue antenatal hypertensive treatment</li><li>See **Epidural anaesthesia** guideline – **Investigations**</li><li>If BP stable <150 mmHg systolic, do not routinely limit duration of second stage of labour</li></ul>	<ul><li>BP continuously</li><li>Continue antenatal hypertensive treatment</li><li>If BP controlled <150 mmHg systolic, do not routinely limit duration of second stage of labour</li><li>If BP does not respond to initial treatment, advise operative birth</li></ul>

Postnatal care

- See **Postnatal care** above

Recurrence risk and long-term health risks

- Women who experienced gestational hypertension risk developing:
- gestational hypertension in future pregnancy ranges from about 1 in 6 (16%) pregnancies to about 1 in 2 (47%) pregnancies
- pre-eclampsia in future pregnancy ranges from 1 in 50 (2%) to about 1 in 14 (7%) pregnancies

Long-term health risks of cardiovascular disease

- Women who have experienced gestational hypertension or pre-eclampsia have an increased risk of developing hypertension and its complications in later life

Long-term risk of end-stage kidney disease

- Inform women with a history of hypertension without proteinuria and no hypertension at the postnatal review (6–8 weeks after delivery) that although the relative risk of end-stage kidney disease is increased, the absolute risk is low and no further follow-up is necessary

GESTATIONAL HYPERTENSION WITH PROTEINURIA (PRE-ECLAMPSIA)

Introduction

- Once a diagnosis of pre-eclampsia is made, risk of maternal and perinatal mortality and morbidity is increased (see **Severe pre-eclampsia** guideline)
- Clinical management is often determined by drawing a balance between maternal and fetal considerations. For example, the timing of birth depends on mother's condition and risk of intrauterine death of baby or, if born, neonatal death or morbidity as a result of prematurity

Antenatal care (see Antihypertensive treatment and prenatal counselling above)

Mild hypertension (BP 140/90–149/99 mmHg)	Moderate hypertension (BP 150/100–159/109 mmHg)	Severe hypertension (BP ≥160/110 mmHg)
● Do not treat hypertension ● Measure BP at least 4 times a day ● Test kidney function, electrolytes, FBC, LFT twice a week	● Treat with first-line oral labetalol to keep BP <150/80–100 mmHg ● Measure BP at least 4 times a day ● Test kidney function, electrolytes, FBC, LFT 3 times a week	● Urgent referral to hospital ● Obstetric middle grade obstetrician (ST3–7 or equivalent e.g. staff grade, clinical fellow) or consultant assessment ● Consultant obstetrician as lead professional ● Treat with first-line oral labetalol to keep BP <150/80–100 mmHg ● Measure BP >4 times daily depending on clinical circumstances ● Test kidney function, electrolytes, FBC, LFT 3 times a week ● VTE risk assessment

Timing of birth

Before 34 weeks

- Manage conservatively until 34 weeks
- Obstetric consultant or middle grade obstetrician (ST3–7 or equivalent e.g. staff grade, clinical fellow) to assess daily to review management plan
- If delivery likely before 35 weeks' gestation, give corticosteroids
- Offer birth (after discussion with neonatologist and anaesthetist) if:
- severe refractory hypertension
- maternal or fetal clinical condition deteriorates

34–36+6 weeks

- If required course of corticosteroids completed, recommend birth after 34 weeks if pre-eclampsia with severe hypertension
- If pre-eclampsia with mild or moderate hypertension, offer birth at 34–36+6 weeks depending on maternal and fetal condition, risk factors and availability of neonatal intensive care

After 37+0 weeks

- Recommend birth within 24–48 hr

Fetal monitoring

- Ultrasound for fetal growth and amniotic fluid volume. Umbilical artery Doppler velocimetry at diagnosis if conservative management planned
- Do not repeat more than every 2 weeks
- EFM at diagnosis. Repeat if change in fetal movement reported by woman, vaginal bleeding, abdominal pain, deterioration in maternal condition

Intrapartum care

- Mild and moderate hypertension (140/90–159/109 mmHg)
- measure BP hourly
- continue antenatal hypertensive treatment
- carry out haematological and biochemical monitoring according to criteria from antenatal period
- If BP stable, do not routinely limit duration of second stage of labour

Postnatal care

● See **Postnatal care** above

Haematological and biochemical monitoring

● In women who have pre-eclampsia with mild or moderate hypertension or after step-down from critical care:

○ measure platelet count, LFT and serum creatinine 48–72 hr after birth or step-down

○ if results are normal at 48–72 hr, do not repeat platelet count, transaminases or serum creatinine measurement

● If biochemical and haematological indices are improving but stay within the abnormal range in women with pre-eclampsia who have given birth, repeat platelet count, LFT and serum creatinine measurement as clinically indicated and at postnatal review (6–8 weeks after birth)

● If biochemical and haematological indices are not improving relative to pregnancy ranges in women with pre-eclampsia who have given birth, repeat platelet count, LFT and serum creatinine measurement as clinically indicated

● In women with pre-eclampsia who have given birth, carry out a urinary reagent-strip test at the postnatal review (6–8 weeks after birth)

● In women who had pre-eclampsia and still have proteinuria (1+ or more) at postnatal review (6–8 weeks after birth), offer a further review at 3 months after birth to assess kidney function and consider referral for specialist renal assessment

Issue 3
Issued: April 2015
Expires: April 2017

DEFINITION

Artificially initiate uterine contractions leading to progressive dilatation and effacement of the cervix and delivery of baby. Includes women with intact membranes and those with spontaneous rupture of membranes but who are not in labour

INDICATIONS

Prevention of prolonged pregnancy (term plus 10–14 days)

- Ultrasound at <20 weeks to confirm gestation and reduce need for induction for perceived post-term pregnancy
- In uncomplicated pregnancies, offer induction of labour between term plus 10–14 days
- Prolonged pregnancy >41 weeks
- Pre-labour ruptured of membranes (>37 weeks' gestation) – see **Pre-labour rupture of membranes** guideline

Other (this list is not exhaustive)

- Diabetes
- Hypertension
- Growth restriction
- Antepartum haemorrhage (APH)
- Multiple pregnancy
- Cholestasis
- Previous stillbirth

Maternal request <41 weeks' gestation

- Consider when compelling psychological or social reasons and woman has favourable cervix (Bishop's score ≥5) and resources allow. Refer to a consultant clinic

PREGNANCY BEYOND 42 WEEKS' GESTATION

- Advise women choosing to continue pregnancy beyond 42 weeks, despite adequate explanation of risks, to closely monitor fetal movement pattern and refer to obstetric consultant for plan of care
  - ultrasound estimation of maximum amniotic pool depth
  - umbilical artery Doppler study
  - electronic fetal monitoring (EFM)

METHODS OF INDUCTION OF LABOUR

Membrane sweeping

Not recommended if membranes have ruptured

- Before considering other methods for induction, offer membrane sweep according to local practice. This has been shown to increases probability of labour starting naturally within 48 hr
- May be carried out in woman's home, antenatal clinic or hospital

Midwife/doctor will:

- Provide full explanation of procedure
- Obtain and record consent
- Inform woman that membrane sweeping is not associated with an increase in maternal or neonatal infection but the procedure can result in increased levels of discomfort and bleeding
- Provide 'Induction of labour' leaflet (if available locally)
- Ensure woman has relevant contact telephone numbers

MEDICAL INDUCTION OF LABOUR

- In nulliparous or multiparous women with intact membranes with unfavourable cervix, use prostaglandin in preference to oxytocin
- In nulliparous or multiparous women with ruptured membranes regardless of cervical status, prostaglandin or oxytocin are equally effective in induction of labour

Nulliparous women	Multiparous women

● Administer first dose prostaglandin:
  2 mg gel **or**
  3 mg tablet **or**
  10 mg Dinoprostone (Propess) pessary
  (times will be unit specific)
	● Administer first dose prostaglandin
	  1 mg gel **or**
	  3 mg tablet **or**
	  10 mg Dinoprostone (Propess) pessary
	  (times will be unit specific)

● Midwife will perform vaginal examination to assess state of cervix, whether contracting or not:

6 hr after initial dose of gel or tablet

24 hr after initial dose of Dinoprostone (Propess) pessary

● If, at next examination, artificial rupture of membranes (ARM) is possible, perform regardless of Bishop's score

● If ARM not possible, administer second dose but withhold if woman is contracting regularly, painfully and palpably

For primips, maximum dose of prostaglandin is 3 mg gel, 6 mg tablet or 10 mg Dinoprostone (Propess) pessary in 24 hr

For multips, maximum dose of prostaglandin is 2 mg gel, 6 mg tablet or 10 mg Dinoprostone (Propess) pessary in 24 hr

Contraindications to induction of labour with prostaglandin

● Sensitivity to prostaglandins

● Clinical suspicion or definite evidence of pre-existing fetal distress

● Uncontrolled asthmatic

● Contraindications to vaginal birth e.g. uncontrolled severe pre-eclampsia, mechanical obstruction to delivery, placenta praevia

Relative contraindications

● Previous caesarean section – see **Vaginal birth after caesarean section** guideline

● Predisposition to uterine rupture

● Acute cervicitis and vaginitis

Inducability rating (modified Bishop's score)
For the purpose of this guideline modified Bishop's score is used to assess cervical condition

Cervical feature	Pelvic score (circle appropriate number)			
	0	1	2	3
Cervix position	Post	Centre	Anterior	–
Consistency	Firm	Medium	Soft	–
Length (cm)	3	2	1	0
Dilatation (cm)	0	1–2	3–4	5+
Station* to spines	-3	-2	-1	0+

*Station is measured in cm relative to ischial spines

Issue 3
Issued: April 2015
Expires: April 2017

OXYTOCIN

● After artificial rupture of membranes or spontaneous rupture of membranes, discuss commencement of oxytocin with woman and obstetric medical staff – see **Oxytocin** guideline for dose regimen

> *Do not begin oxytocin infusion until 6 hr elapsed following administration of prostaglandin gel or tablets or 30 min after removal of Dinoprostone (Propess) pessary*

ANTENATAL MANAGEMENT AND BOOKING OF PLANNED INDUCTION OF LABOUR (LOW-RISK PREGNANCIES)

41 weeks

Community midwife/doctor will:

● Perform routine antenatal assessment, to include:
- blood pressure
- urine for proteinuria and glycosuria
- measure fundal height and plot on growth chart
- check position of baby
- auscultate fetal heart and enquire about fetal activity

● Following explanation of the procedure, perform a membrane sweep and inform woman of findings

● Explain she may experience discomfort and the passing of a show and advise to contact maternity unit if she experiences bleeding, spontaneous rupture of membranes, abdominal pain or contraction

● Arrange admission date and time for induction at 40 weeks plus 10–14 days' gestation

● Record all discussions indicating woman's understanding of her plan of care

ADMISSION AND MANAGEMENT OF PROSTAGLANDIN INDUCTION (LOW-RISK PREGNANCIES)

● Admit and perform general observations:
- temperature
- pulse
- blood pressure
- respiratory rate and document MEWS score
- repeat in accordance with Unit guidance
- urinalysis
- full antenatal examination

● Obtain and review full history, confirm gestation and reason for induction and carry out:
- abdominal examination to determine lie and fifths of the head palpable in the abdomen
- fetal heart assessment

● Give woman information regarding discomfort associated with procedure and pain relief options

● Explain there is no association with an increase in maternal or neonatal infection, bleeding, contractions and hyperstimulation

● Obtain consent

● Perform external EFM for 20 min to confirm fetal wellbeing

● Assess cervix using Bishop's score and record findings

● Administer prostaglandin as per local guidance

● Advise woman to remain recumbent for 30–60 min

- Provided initial monitoring on admission is within normal parameters, reassess fetal wellbeing:

- EFM trace of 20 min once contractions have commenced

- discontinue EFM after 20 min providing fetal heart remains within normal parameters

- If, at any time throughout the procedure, fetal heart rate is outside normal parameters, continue EFM and inform middle grade obstetrician (ST3–7 or equivalent e.g. staff grade, clinical fellow) or consultant

- Encourage woman to mobilise freely and consider using non-pharmacological pain relief/simple analgesia

Uterine hypercontractility with prostaglandin

- In the presence of abnormal fetal heart rate patterns and uterine hypercontractility, consider administration of subcutaneous terbutaline 250 microgram

ANTENATAL MANAGEMENT OF PLANNED INDUCTION OF LABOUR (HIGH-RISK PREGNANCIES)

- Consultant obstetrician will be lead professional for all cases

- Obstetric medical staff will decide place of induction (routine maternal wards are not appropriate in certain circumstances e.g. vaginal birth after caesarean section)

- Obstetric medical staff will determine frequency of maternal and fetal observations required over and above those for low-risk pregnancy

- Discuss plan of care with all high-risk women to decide timing and method of induction of labour

- Provide 'Induction of labour' information leaflet (if available locally)

- Follow procedure in **Low-risk pregnancies**

INDUCTION OF LABOUR WITH A PREVIOUS CAESAREAN SECTION

- The decision to induce a woman with a previous caesarean section should be made by an obstetric consultant following a vaginal examination. Vaginal examination is useful in determining method of induction

- Offer membrane sweeping

- Discuss risks of induction of labour with woman (e.g. failed induction/repeat caesarean section, scar rupture) and document in maternal healthcare record

- risk of scar rupture is approximately doubled with artificial rupture of membranes and oxytocin and increased five-fold with prostaglandin. If both oxytocin and prostaglandin are used the risk is increased 25 times

- With a relatively low modified Bishop's score, consider proceeding directly to artificial rupture of membranes or use of transcervical catheter induction – see **Transcervical catheter induction** guideline

- Discuss and document individualised management plan using local proforma

- For women with a previous caesarean section undergoing induction, insert a cannula and take blood for FBC and group and save

- Inform obstetric anaesthetic middle grade (ST3–7 or equivalent e.g. staff grade, clinical fellow)

- Monitor fetal wellbeing closely throughout

- EFM continuously from the onset of even mild contractions or any pain until delivery

- If only indication for induction is post-term pregnancy, consider monitoring fetal wellbeing beyond 42 weeks' gestation

Issue 3
Issued: April 2015
Expires: April 2017

FAILED INDUCTION OF LABOUR

- If amniotomy still not possible after 2 doses of prostaglandin gel or tablet or 24 hr Dinoprostone (Propess) use, induction of labour has failed

- give third dose of prostaglandin (1 mg gel or 3 mg tablet) or extend Dinoprostone (Propess) use for a further 6 hr

- If amniotomy still not possible, discuss with consultant obstetrician and arrange review

- Discuss the following options with the woman:

- caesarean section

- transcervical catheter induction (if used locally) – see **Transcervical catheter induction** guideline

- abandon process and repeat after an interval i.e. 24 hr

INTRODUCTION

- Unless otherwise stated, this guideline applies to healthy term infants
- Where expressed breast milk (EBM) is mentioned, it refers to mother's own EBM

Antenatal period

- Promote breastfeeding to woman and give information and reassurance regarding newborn infant feeding patterns
- If woman chooses to formula feed, give support and information on safe practices – see **Formula feeding**
- Do not question woman about her choice of feeding method, which can limit further discussion and does not allow for change of mind

SKIN-TO-SKIN CONTACT

- Skin-to-skin contact immediately after birth (following delayed cord clamping) promotes an early feed
- Aim to provide an uninterrupted period of skin-to-skin contact in a quiet environment for one hour, or at least until after first feed
- Ensure mother comfortable and avoid excessive heat-loss in baby
- Never interrupt skin-to-skin contact to perform routine procedures (e.g. weighing baby)
- Where condition of mother or baby requires medical intervention, this will take precedence over immediate skin-to-skin contact
- commence contact once condition of mother and baby stable
- Reassure woman undergoing a caesarean section that skin-to-skin contact will be initiated as soon as possible after birth, in theatre or recovery room, depending on clinical situation
- Document skin-to-skin contact and record reason for any delay in maternal healthcare record

- If mother wishes to end skin-to-skin contact before first breastfeed, advise that ending contact for anything other than a short time may be detrimental to initiation of breastfeeding. Document mother's decision in maternal healthcare record
- Allow mother to transfer to postnatal ward with baby still in skin-to-skin contact

Benefits

- Keeps baby warm
- Promotes bonding
- Helps baby's heartbeat and breathing to settle after birth

POSTNATAL WARD

- Check baby's temperature was normal before transfer
- On admission to postnatal ward, observe colour and general appearance of baby
- If baby is well and not showing signs of wanting to feed, leave alone
- When baby showing feeding cues, offer assistance to breastfeed
- Unless it is necessary, for clinical reasons, to separate mother and baby, mother has primary responsibility for baby's care on postnatal areas. Baby will remain with mother 24 hr/day to allow her to recognise feeding cues (see **Baby-led feeding and feeding cues**) and encourage night-time breastfeeds/formula feeds

> *Do not routinely separate mother and baby at night whether formula-fed, breastfed or delivered by caesarean section*

- If mother requests separation from her baby for 'settling' by staff, explain the benefits of staying close to baby and document decision and length of separation in maternal healthcare record. Return baby to mother as soon as baby settles

Issue 3
Issued: April 2015
Expires: April 2017

BABY-LED FEEDING AND FEEDING CUES

- Ensure mother understands the nature of feeding cues, the importance of quick response (rather than waiting until baby cries) and is aware of normal feeding patterns, including cluster feeding and 'growth spurts'. This is applicable to breast and formula fed babies

- Unless, clinically indicated, encourage baby-led feeding, allowing baby to feed for as long and as often as he/she wants. Where clinical procedures are necessary, they should not interfere with this process

- Observation of the sleepy baby (for either method of feeding) is important to ensure vital signs such as colour, respiration rate, heart rate and temperature are stable and that there are no signs of hypoglycaemia (e.g. following administration of pethidine to mother during labour)

Breastfed babies

- Early and frequent breastfeeding has many benefits including:

- enhances milk supply – the more milk removed from the breast, the more milk the mother will produce

- reduces incidence of physiological jaundice

- Inform mother that it is acceptable to wake baby for feeding if her breasts become overfull. Explain the importance of night-time feeding for milk production

- Length of individual feeds will vary considerably. The length of the feed is determined by the rate of milk transfer from mother to baby. Encourage mother to allow baby to empty the first breast before offering the second

- Babies who are not removed from the breast but allowed to finish a feed spontaneously are more likely to take the high fat hind milk which will encourage satisfaction and weight gain

Formula-fed babies

- After explaining the avoidance of 'over feeding', encourage mothers to feed in the same way taking amounts of milk that the baby wishes at each feed

BREASTFEEDING

- Human milk is important in establishing enteral nutrition

- To promote optimum health benefits, babies should be breastfed exclusively until 6 months of age and should continue to breastfeed until the age of 2 yr

- Frequent feeds during the initial period will help prevent breast engorgement

- Midwife or skilled support worker should be available during mother's hospital stay to assist with breastfeeding

- support should also be available to mothers who choose to deliver at home

Information for mother

- Give mother information on how to obtain advice and support in hospital and at home

- Give verbal and written information on how to recognise effective feeding (UNICEF 'Recognising breastfeeding is going well' tool if available locally). Including signs that baby is receiving sufficient milk and what to do if not

- Recognise when breastfeeding not progressing normally e.g. sore nipples, breast inflammation

Health benefits

Baby	Mother
● Reduced risk of:	● Reduced risk of:
○ gastroenteritis	○ ovarian and breast cancer
○ diarrhoea	○ osteoporosis
○ urinary tract infection	
○ chest infection	
○ ear infection	
○ obesity	
○ diabetes	
○ leukaemia	

Initiating breastfeeding immediately after delivery

- ● Encourage mother to hold baby (skin-to-skin contact) in a calm environment as soon as possible after delivery – see **Skin-to-skin contact**
- ● Midwife will assist with first breastfeed as soon as baby shows interest
- ● following a period of uninterrupted skin-to-skin contact, many babies will self-attach
- ● Early suckling helps promote uterine contraction, facilitating early passage of meconium and baby's blood glucose stabilisation
- ● If first feed not achieved within 4 hr, start active intervention – see **Healthy term baby who is reluctant to feed**

Exclusive breastfeeding/ artificial supplements

- ● Unless it is medically indicated or is parents' fully informed choice, do not give food or drink (including water or artificial feed) other than breast milk to newborn breastfeeding infants
- ● if necessary, for clinical reasons, trained midwife or neonatologist will make the decision to offer supplementary feeds after discussion with parents
- ● Before introducing artificial milk to breastfed babies, encourage mother to express breast milk to be given by feeding cup or syringe to reduce the need for artificial feeds

- ● If supplements of formula are given, provide optimal care and support, and review each feed to ensure:
- ○ minimal formula use
- ○ maximum breast milk use
- ○ support to increase milk production
- ○ cup feeding rather than teat feeding
- ○ support to express and stimulate breasts
- ● This proactive approach will reduce the need to offer artificial feeds and help to support mother's lactation

How to breastfeed and maintain lactation

Correct positioning and attachment

- ● Good positioning and attachment are key to successful breastfeeding It:
- ○ ensures good milk supply and transfer from mother to baby
- ○ prevents sore nipples
- ○ pain-free feeding
- ● Poor positioning and attachment may cause unsettled baby in immediate postpartum period. Assist mother to attach baby to breast correctly
- ● Document assistance given and outcome in appropriate healthcare record

Avoid teats and dummies

- ● Teats and dummies can hinder baby's ability to attach to the breast while learning to breastfeed in the early weeks and can interfere with baby-led feeding

Issue 3
Issued: April 2015
Expires: April 2017

Assessment

- Midwife will assess breastfeeding within first 48 hr and again on or around day 5 to determine whether effective milk transfer is taking place and if further support required
- Document findings using your local breastfeeding assessment tool
- If assessment indicates a potential feeding problem, observe a full breastfeed and document
- If mother experiences difficulty breastfeeding, refer immediately to midwife/breastfeeding specialist or neonatal team for further assessment, support and plan of care

Expressing breast milk

- It is important that mothers understand why and when hand-expressing is useful
- **In hospital:** As routine, before transfer home, teach mother to hand-express breast milk and, if available locally, give information leaflet
- **Home birth:** Instruct mother as soon as possible after birth
- Offer a visit by community staff

Preterm/sick baby

- Encourage mothers who are separated from their babies to begin expressing milk as soon as possible after birth as early initiation has long-term benefits for milk production

- Neonatal nurse caring for baby, and mother's midwife will show mother how to express milk by hand and by pump
- If available locally, give mothers the 'How to express your breast milk' leaflet
- If baby very preterm or very low birth weight, more frequent expressing is advised (8–12 times in 24 hr)
- If baby known to be at risk of developing hypoglycaemia is receiving care on the postnatal ward, midwife responsible for mother and baby will assist in initiating and maintaining lactation
- practical care and help may be delegated to a skilled maternity support worker or healthcare assistant, but the overall responsibility remains with the midwife
- See also the following guidelines:
- **Promotion, initiation and maintenance of lactation in the mother of a preterm or sick infant** guideline (if available locally)
- **Breastfeeding** guideline, **Breast milk expression** guideline, **Breast milk handling and storage** guideline and **Hypoglycaemia** guideline in the Staffordshire, Shropshire & Black Country Newborn and Maternity Network Neonatal guidelines (if used locally)

Reasons why baby may not get enough breast milk (Note: several factors may contribute in any one situation)

Factors related to breastfeeding	Other factors	Factors occasionally associated with breast milk insufficiency	Factors rarely associated with breast milk insufficiency
• Delayed start in breastfeeding • Inefficient suckling • Infrequent feeds • Scheduled feeds • Short feeds • Supplementary feeds • Use of a teat • Use of a dummy	• Lack of confidence in mother, either by herself or those around her (indirectly) • Tiredness, stress, worry (indirectly)	• Dislike of breastfeeding (indirectly) • Medication (e.g. contraceptive pill, diuretics) • Pregnancy • Alcohol/smoking • Prematurity, illness/abnormality in baby	• Retained products of conception • Rejection of baby • Severe malnutrition • Inadequate breast development

Assessment of breastfeeding

At each postnatal visit/check

Abnormal findings trigger further action, see **Table** below

Baby	Breasts	Breastfeeding
● Jaundiced and sleepy or difficult to rouse for feeding ● Feeding <8 times in 24 hr and/or not sustaining effective suckling pattern ● Feeding very frequently i.e. consistently >12 times in 24 hr ● Consistently feeding for >45 min or <5 min ● Unsettled after or during feed	● Engorgement or mastitis ● Trauma to nipples: ○ nipples misshapen or 'pinched' at end of feeds ● Breasts not filling/ draining as expected	● Difficult attachment ● No change in sucking pattern i.e. from initial rapid sucks with pauses and audible swallows ● Baby 'fussy' at breast e.g. on and off the breast frequently during feed or refusing to breastfeed

HEALTHY TERM BABY WHO IS RELUCTANT TO FEED

● Hypoglycaemia is unlikely to be problematic in healthy, term, well grown babies. These babies are low risk and routine blood glucose monitoring is unnecessary

● There is no evidence that long intervals between feeds in the first 24 hr will adversely affect healthy term newborns

● Some babies will feed <4 times in the first 24 hr. At least 3–4 feeds are expected in this period increasing to 8–12 thereafter in any 24 hr period

● Encourage healthy term babies to breastfeed in the first hour after birth, preferably on delivery suite or, if not, when baby is ready

● Some babies may not be keen to feed soon after delivery

● Encourage skin-to-skin contact between mother and baby (see **Skin-to-skin contact**)

● Encourage baby-led feeding from birth (see **Baby-led feeding and feeding cues**)

● Assist mother to initiate breastfeeding

Artificial teats, dummies and nipple shields

● **Discourage the use of** artificial teats or dummies to breastfeeding babies during the establishment of breastfeeding. If a breastfed baby seems unsettled, it is more important to assess carefully and, if necessary, improve mother's feeding technique

● If parents wish to use teats, dummies or nipple shields, advise that dummies may have a detrimental effect on breastfeeding and lactation (UNICEF UK 2008). Document discussion and parent(s) decision in postnatal record

● If baby requires additional fluids, give these by cup rather than by bottle to avoid nipple/teat confusion and encourage baby to develop correct tongue technique. Offering bottles may encourage baby to develop a preference for a teat

Issue 3
Issued: April 2015
Expires: April 2017

- **Nipple shields** are not recommended except in extreme circumstances and then only for as short a time as possible. Explain the disadvantages to mother before commencing use:
- nipple soreness caused by incorrect positioning and attachment
- difficulty in improving positioning and attachment
- reduced milk transfer to baby
- increased risk of mastitis and breast abscess
- If used, mother must be supervised by a skilled practitioner and given assistance to discontinue use as soon as possible

SUPPLEMENTATION

Medical indications for formula supplementation

- Each baby and situation will be individually assessed. Indications include:
- low birth weight <1500 g
- metabolic disorders e.g. galactosaemia, maple syrup urine disease, PKU
- very preterm e.g. <32 weeks' gestation
- at risk of hypoglycaemia e.g. preterm, small for gestational age, intrapartum stress, illness or maternal diabetes – if blood glucose fails to respond to optimal breastfeeding in spite of frequent effective suckling
- persistent faltering growth/significant weight loss/hypernatraemia
- HIV positive mother – see **HIV positive women** guideline
- cytotoxic chemotherapy
- certain medications e.g. iodine, and drugs that cause drowsiness
- active herpes on breast
- breast abscess where there is pus coming from the nipple
- See **Breastfeeding** guideline and **Abstinence syndrome** guideline in the Staffordshire, Shropshire & Black Country Newborn and Maternity Network Neonatal guidelines (if used locally)

- When breastfeeding is temporarily delayed or interrupted, assist mother in establishing and maintaining lactation e.g. through manual or hand pump expression of milk, in preparation for resumption of breastfeeding

Documentation

- Record the following in maternal healthcare record:
- discussions with parent(s) and informed consent obtained
- reason for administering supplements, whether for clinical reasons or parents' request
- supplements used
- Complete appropriate formula audit form (if used locally) and send to breastfeeding co-ordinator

Baby has breastfed at delivery

Within 6 hr of birth

- Offer assistance with second breastfeed and document
- If baby sleeping or unwilling to feed, try again in 2 hr or earlier if baby shows signs of hunger/wakefulness

Baby has not fed since birth

At 4 hr

- Check heart rate, temperature, respiration rate, tone, colour and baby's general appearance again. If baby appears well and is still reluctant to feed, gently stimulate by:
- unwrapping
- resuming skin-to-skin contact
- gentle massage
- tempt at the breast
- Encourage mother to hand-express colostrum and give via cup/syringe (use of a breast pump is unlikely to obtain any colostrum and may cause nipple trauma)

- Review baby 2-hrly and repeat above process until baby has successfully breastfed
- Document all care given on a feeding chart

Baby not taken feed by 12 hr

- If baby refuses to breastfeed, is unable to cup feed, or no colostrum available, midwife to assess baby to determine whether neonatal referral necessary
- Midwife/neonatologist and mother will formulate an individualised care plan
- If baby will not accept cup or small syringe feeds, partnership decision-making with neonatal medical colleagues is recommended to establish why and agree management plan. Explain suggested care plan to mother
- If baby is otherwise well and clinical signs are stable, blood glucose testing is not routinely helpful
- low risk babies can mobilise alternative fuels like ketones as an energy source in the presence of low glucose
- Encourage mother to express milk 8 times in 24 hr, (including during the night) and give colostrum, when available, via cup or syringe or by direct expression into baby's mouth
- Stop monitoring temperature, respirations, heart rate and muscle tone once baby is feeding regularly and neonatal/midwifery staff are happy with progress
- Use feeding chart to assess whether feeding is established for a minimum of 24 hr
- Observe a breastfeed to ensure correct positioning and attachment and take a thorough breastfeeding history

> *Reluctance to feed may be the only sign of a sick baby. Consider the possibility of septicaemia or inborn errors of metabolism. Careful clinical surveillance is key to management*

Amount not increasing

- If, after 12 hr, amount of colostrum only 'droplets', support mother and attempt to allay anxiety, which is helpful in establishing colostrum/milk flow by the natural release of oxytocin
- It would be valuable to increase expressing frequency from 8 to 10–12 times in 24 hr to ensure more stimulation of breasts and increased amounts given to baby
- Explain carefully to mother the rationale for temporarily increasing expressing frequency
- Ensure mother is hand-expressing and using the pump effectively and safely
- All colostrum expressed must be given to baby
- Observe breastfeeding attempts and encourage skin-to-skin contact as much as possible in a dimly lit quiet environment
- Complete feed chart until breastfeeding established and record baby's urine and stool output. Report any deviations from normal to neonatal medical staff

Breastfed baby 'sleepy' or 'reluctant to feed' in second 24 hr of life

- Refer to the neonatal team for assessment
- Ensure there are no anatomical reasons preventing breastfeeding attachment e.g. cleft palate/tongue tie/ mother's breast or nipple anatomy
- Keep baby close to mother – skin-to-skin contact
- Provide emotional reassurance and support for mother
- Ensure mother understands feeding cues and is trying at every opportunity to breastfeed
- Observe and assess a full breastfeed, and offer breastfeeding support where necessary
- Avoid teats and dummies

- Continue to express and cup feed colostrum frequently
- Maintain feed chart until breastfeeding established
- Record plan (agreed with mother, midwife and neonatal team) in maternal healthcare record/neonatal notes
- Review progress with mother 12-hrly, ensuring baby has at least 8–12 feeds in this time period
- Observe wet and dirty nappies
- Consider biological nurturing positions

Assessment of output

- At each postnatal visit, enquire about baby's output, together with ongoing monitoring by mother
  - inadequate output (less than that specified – see **Table** below) triggers weight assessment and implementation of appropriate management plan
- The following findings are 'reassuring' in a breastfed baby. Any deviation from this should trigger further assessment

Age	Day 1–2	Day 3–4	Day 5–6	Day 7–28 and beyond
Urine Number of wet nappies per day	1–2 or more Urates may be present*	≥3 Nappies feel heavier	≥5	≥6 heavy
Stools Number per day, colour, consistency	≥1 Dark green/black 'tarlike' (meconium)	≥2 Change in colour and consistency - brown/green/yellow becoming looser ('changing stool')	≥2 Yellow May be quite watery	≥2 At least size of £2 coin, yellow and watery, 'seedy' appearance

* Urates are normal bladder discharges in the first few days but persistent urates may indicate insufficient milk intake
- After 28 days, baby will establish own frequency of passing stools - may pass several per day or have several days' gap between

FORMULA FEEDING

Early postnatal period

- Encourage mother to hold baby in a calm environment as soon as possible after delivery – see **Skin-to-skin contact**
- Explain how mother may obtain help with feeding while in hospital
- Ensure mother is supported with feeding until she feels confident
- Document formula feeding progress and all information given on the feeding care plan, and maternal healthcare record

Sterilising equipment

- Equipment that is used to store formula or feed an infant must be kept very clean
- Discuss with parents and offer the following information:
  - wash milk-related feeding equipment thoroughly in hot soapy water, using a clean brush inside and out (especially the rim), before sterilising, until baby is 1 yr old
  - rinse well in clean water after washing
  - check equipment regularly for signs of deterioration. If any doubt, throw away

Technique

- **Boiling (saucepan)** – all equipment must be under the water level of the pan, with no air bubbles trapped inside
- Do not allow the pan to boil dry

- Boil for at least 10 min
- Keep pan covered with a lid until equipment is used
- **Steam or microwave sterilisers** – follow manufacturer's instructions
- **Chemical sterilisation** (tablets or fluid) – follow manufacturer's instructions
- Ensure all equipment is under the fluid – with no trapped air bubbles – a plunger or plate can be used to keep items under water
- leave submersed for at least 30 min or as per manufacturer's instructions
- Always wash hands before removing equipment from the steriliser
- Make a fresh solution every 24 hr
- Rinse equipment with cool boiled water

Formula milk preparation/ storage

- Discuss with parent(s) and give leaflets on bottle feeding
- Demonstrate technique in early postnatal period before discharge home and, if necessary, again in the home environment. Document in maternal healthcare record
- Wash, rinse and dry hands thoroughly
- Use a clean work surface
- Use boiled tap water that has been left to cool for a few minutes (<30 min – it should still be >70ºC) – to reduce the risk of growth of bacteria found in infant formula powder
- Remind parents **not to use** bottled water due to variable mineral content
- **Make up a fresh bottle for each feed,** following preparation instructions on tin

> *Storing prepared formula milk increases the risk of bacterial growth (powdered infant formula is not sterile)*

- If using cold water sterilisation, rinse feeding equipment with cooled boiled water (not water straight from tap), or shake solution off well

- Add powder using only the scoop provided with the tin – level off with a plastic knife or spatula (one scoop of powder to 30 mL of water)
- Fill bottle to required mark – always water first before powder
- Place the disc, teat and cap onto bottle, and shake well until all powder has dissolved
- To cool the milk, hold bottle, with cap covering teat, under cold running water.
- Remind parents to check temperature of feed on inner wrist before giving to baby
- After feeding, throw away any unused milk
- Freshly prepared powdered formula milk will keep for 2 hr at room temperature, after which time, discard

How to bottle-feed

- Hold baby upright with head supported in a comfortable neutral position (twisted neck makes swallowing difficult)
- To start the feed, brush the teat against baby's lips. Baby will open mouth with tongue down, which helps draw the teat in
- Keep teat full of milk, to avoid intake of air
- Hold bottle horizontal to the ground, tilting just enough to ensure baby is taking milk
- Babies feed in bursts of sucking with short pauses. In this position the milk will stop flowing when baby pauses – allowing baby to rest
- There should be bubbles in the bottle as baby feeds, if not, break the suction – you should see bubbles rushing back into the remaining milk
- Babies may need short breaks during the feed and may need to be winded
- Discuss baby-led feeding – babies may take different amounts at different times – and the tin provides a guide only

- Advise parents not to try to give more milk at one feed in the hope baby will go longer before needing another feed. If baby is given more milk than necessary, he/she is likely to gain too much weight, or be sick

- Discuss feeding cues with parents so that they can recognise when their baby is hungry and encourage parents to stay close to baby in order to recognize these cues

- Encourage parents to hold baby close for feeding, offering eye contact. Skin-to-skin contact can be enjoyed

- As with breastfeeding, bottle feeding is a social interaction, not just for delivering nutrition. Aim to keep number of people feeding baby to a minimum

- **Never** leave baby alone with a bottle

Feeding away from home

- It is safest to carry a measured amount of milk powder in a small clean and dry container, a flask of hot water that has been boiled and an empty sterilised feeding bottle

- Bottle must be cooled before feeding

- If the above is not possible, the feed can be prepared at home and cooled at the back of the fridge. Take out of fridge before leaving home and carry in a cool bag with an ice pack. Use within 4 hr or, if destination reached within 4 hr, store at back of fridge

- Never store feeds for >24 hr. It is always safer to make up a fresh bottle

- Ready-to-drink, formula milk is an alternative

Formula-fed baby who is reluctant to feed

- Encourage skin-to-skin contact to stimulate feeding cue

- Offer frequent opportunities to feed

- If unwilling to suck from teat – try cup feeding

- small volumes in first two days is normal

- Clinically assess baby at 12 hr (colour, tone, behaviour, temperature, respiration, heart rate). If concerns, seek neonatal team assessment

- If baby not waking for feeds or sucking eagerly at the bottle by 36–48 hr, request neonatal team assessment

- Alternative feeding methods may be required based on clinical indication

DISCHARGE AND FOLLOW-UP

Before discharge home

Rooming in

- Explain and encourage parents to stay close to baby, sharing the same room for first six months of life

- Ensure parent(s) are aware of the appropriate age for introducing complimentary foods

Breastfed baby	Formula-fed baby
● Give mother:	● Complete bottle-feeding checklist
verbal and written information about local support groups, including contact details for voluntary breastfeeding counsellors, 24 hr national help lines including National Breastfeeding helpline, the Breastfeeding Network, National Childbirth Trust, La Leche League and Association of Breastfeeding Mothers	● Offer demonstration of sterilisation of equipment and reconstitution
	● Document in postnatal section of mother's healthcare plan
	● Mothers who do not wish this, or request early transfer home before it can be arranged should at least be knowledge-able in the preparation, administration and storage of formula milk
● Ensure breastfeeding mothers:	
know how to recognise signs that baby is receiving sufficient milk, and what to do if this is not the case	give 'Bottle feeding' leaflet and 'A guide to infant formula for parents who are bottle feeding' leaflet if available
know how to recognise signs that breastfeeding is not progressing normally (e.g. sore nipples, breast inflammation)	● Where English is not the first language, seek assistance from an interpreter to ensure effective demonstration/discussion
are confident with positioning and attaching baby for breastfeeding	● Translated leaflets are available

● Ensure mother understands feeding cues and the importance of responding, and awareness of normal feeding patterns, including 'cluster feeding' and 'growth spurts'

● Provide written and verbal information on what constitutes healthy newborn behaviour and the signs that should cause concern

● Advise mother to seek help urgently if baby is sleepy and reluctant to feed, after discharge home. Give midwives' contact numbers (24 hr/7 days), infant feeding co-ordinator, breastfeeding support workers, and other professional support

● Home support is provided by community midwives, and breastfeeding support workers

● Further telephone support is available evenings, nights and weekends from maternity unit. While no evening home visits can be undertaken, if the problem is urgent, hospital staff have the discretion to invite mother to attend the ward for assessment and help

● In order to identify potential difficulties, at each contact, healthcare professional will ask about the progress of breastfeeding and assess adequacy of milk transfer within the first 48 hr and on (or around) day 5 using local breastfeeding assessment form – see assessment tool www.babyfriendly.org.uk

Support in the community

● Community midwives will check and reinforce learning

● Ensure particular care and planning so that mothers who begin breastfeeding but later change to formula feeding are given full support to breastfeed while they are doing so, but are provided with appropriate information about formula feeding when decision to change or combine is made

● Healthcare professionals and trained support workers will further instruct on expressing milk, explaining the importance of prevention and management of engorgement and mastitis

● If breastfeeding difficulties present, look for causal factors e.g. tongue tie, cleft palate

Re-admission to hospital with feeding problems within first 28 days

● Follow local follow-up process

Issue 3
Issued: April 2015
Expires: April 2017

Flowchart: Management of breastfeeding in healthy term babies

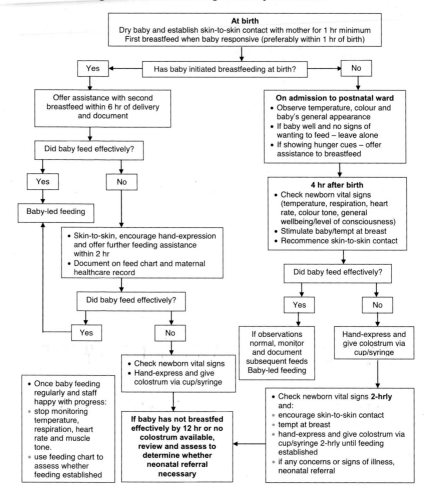

At birth
Dry baby and establish skin-to-skin contact with mother for 1 hr minimum
First breastfeed when baby responsive (preferably within 1 hr of birth)

Has baby initiated breastfeeding at birth?

Yes → Offer assistance with second breastfeed within 6 hr of delivery and document

Did baby feed effectively?

- **Yes** → Baby-led feeding
- **No** → • Skin-to-skin, encourage hand-expression and offer further feeding assistance within 2 hr
  • Document on feed chart and maternal healthcare record

Did baby feed effectively?

- **Yes**
- **No** → • Check newborn vital signs
  • Hand-express and give colostrum via cup/syringe

If baby has not breastfed effectively by 12 hr or no colostrum available, review and assess to determine whether neonatal referral necessary

- Once baby feeding regularly and staff happy with progress:
  - stop monitoring temperature, respiration, heart rate and muscle tone.
  - use feeding chart to assess whether feeding established

No → **On admission to postnatal ward**
- Observe temperature, colour and baby's general appearance
- If baby well and no signs of wanting to feed – leave alone
- If showing hunger cues – offer assistance to breastfeed

4 hr after birth
- Check newborn vital signs (temperature, respiration, heart rate, colour tone, general wellbeing/level of consciousness)
- Stimulate baby/tempt at breast
- Recommence skin-to-skin contact

Did baby feed effectively?

- **Yes** → If observations normal, monitor and document subsequent feeds Baby-led feeding
- **No** → Hand-express and give colostrum via cup/syringe

- Check newborn vital signs **2-hrly** and:
  - encourage skin-to-skin contact
  - tempt at breast
  - hand-express and give colostrum via cup/syringe 2-hrly until feeding established
  - if any concerns or signs of illness, neonatal referral

DEFINITION

- The interval monitoring of fetal heart using Doppler ultrasound or Pinnards

Who

- Advise women who do not have the following maternal, fetal or intrapartum risk factors to have baby's heart monitored by intermittent auscultation
- If risk factors present or structured intermittent auscultation not possible, use continuous electronic fetal monitoring (EFM) – see **Electronic fetal monitoring** guideline

Contraindications

Maternal

- Previous caesarean section/uterine scar
- Pre-eclampsia/eclampsia
- Antepartum haemorrhage
- Prolonged rupture of membranes >24 hr
- Prolonged pregnancy >42 weeks
- Diabetes or other significant medical disorders
- Raised blood pressure (see **Hypertension** guideline)
- Labour with oxytocin
- Abdominal pain
- Trauma/after a fall/RTA
- Cholestasis
- Previous stillbirth or early neonatal death
- Abnormality on auscultation (abnormal baseline, decelerations)

Fetal

- Intrauterine growth restriction/abnormal Doppler
- Prematurity
- Oligohydramnios/polyhydramnios
- Multiple pregnancy
- Breech presentation
- Iso-immunisation
- Suspicious antenatal EFM
- Reduced fetal movements >26 weeks' gestation

How

- Start intermittent auscultation as soon as labour is established
- Auscultate fetal heart using Doppler ultrasound or stethoscope whilst palpating maternal pulse to differentiate between maternal and fetal heart rates (FHR)
- Listen for one full minute after a contraction and record average rate
  - in first stage – at least every 15 min
  - in second stage – at least every 5 min
- Document maternal and fetal heart rates in maternal healthcare record
- Note any intrapartum events that may affect the FHR contemporaneously (at the same time) in maternal healthcare record, sign and note time
- If any concern about decelerations, palpate maternal pulse to differentiate the two heart beats

Electronic fetal monitoring

- Transfer to EFM if:
  - intermittent auscultation is not possible
  - significant meconium-stained liquor (and consider if light meconium staining) – see **Meconium stained liquor** guideline
  - abnormal FHR: ≤100 beats/min or ≥160 beats/min or any decelerations after a contraction
  - maternal pyrexia: 38.0°C once or 37.5°C on two occasions 2 hr apart
  - fresh bleeding developing in labour
  - confirmed delay in first or second stage of labour (see **Delay in labour** guideline)
  - oxytocin use for augmentation
  - epidural analgesia
  - woman's request

DEFINITION	
Latent phase	● Period of time, not necessarily continuous, where there are painful contractions and some cervical change up to 4 cm dilatation – see **Latent phase of labour** guideline
First stage	● Regular painful uterine contractions and progressive cervical dilatation from 4 cm (NICE 2007)
Second stage	**Passive** ● Full dilatation of cervix before or in the absence of expulsive contractions **Active** ● Expulsive contractions with full dilatation of cervical os ● Presenting part of baby visible or active maternal effort in the absence of expulsive contractions
Third stage	● Time of birth of baby to expulsion of placenta and membranes – see **Third stage of labour** guideline

ADVICE TO WOMAN AT ONSET OF LABOUR

● Advise woman to telephone nearest labour ward for advice

● **If homebirth** planned, community midwife will attend

● **If in-patient birth** planned, advise woman to attend the unit for assessment if:

◉ contraction pattern suggesting established labour

◉ history suggestive of rupture of membranes

◉ woman was advised during antenatal period to present early in labour

INITIAL ASSESSMENT OF LABOUR

● In all clinical settings and in all women, midwife must perform a thorough assessment

● If possible, review clinical records before admission, especially with regard to any safeguarding concerns and anaesthetic and neonatal alerts

● Take history

● Assess emotional and physical needs

> *All staff must introduce themselves, greet the woman courteously with a smile and include her in all discussions about her care*

Maternal observations

● Perform the following observations and document on a MEWS chart:

◉ maternal pulse

◉ blood pressure

◉ temperature

◉ respiratory rate

◉ urinalysis

Examination

● Abdominal palpation

◉ fundal height in centimetres

◉ lie

◉ presentation and position

◉ engagement

● Vaginal loss:

◉ liquor colour (e.g. clear or meconium)

◉ show

◉ blood loss and amount

Vaginal assessment

● If in established labour, offer vaginal assessment

◉ explain reason and what is involved

◉ obtain verbal consent

Fetal wellbeing

- Auscultate fetal heart rate (FHR) for a minimum of one full minute immediately after a contraction
- Palpate maternal pulse rate to differentiate between maternal and FHR
- If there is a clinical indication, perform, electronic fetal monitoring (EFM) see **Electronic fetal monitoring** guideline
- Once labour diagnosed, complete intrapartum risk assessment and devise individualised management plan

Pain assessment

- Discuss pain relief options, including woman's choice for coping

Blood and blood products

- If not already done, ask woman if she is prepared to accept blood or blood products – see **Refusing blood and blood products** guideline
- document discussion and woman's decision in maternal healthcare record

Thromboembolism

- Carry out VTE risk assessment using local protocol

Communication and documentation

- Document findings of vaginal assessment
- Discuss findings, birth plan and analgesia with woman and her partner

CLINICAL RISK ASSESSMENT

- Must be performed in all women by a midwife in all clinical settings, whether in maternity unit or at home
- If an obstetrician is involved in woman's care, he/she should repeat risk assessment

Full risk assessment

- Determine level of risk based on:
- medical comorbidity
- anaesthetic history
- previous obstetric history
- lifestyle history
- any concerns with this pregnancy e.g. IUGR
- examination
- observations
- current complaint

Identified risks

- To minimise risk to mother and baby, instigate a management plan for each risk identified
- If risk is such that midwifery-led care is no longer appropriate, discuss with middle grade obstetrician (ST3–7 or equivalent e.g. staff grade, clinical fellow) and transfer care to obstetric team
- Advice for management can also be obtained from resident anaesthetist

> *Assess risk status continuously and change management plan accordingly*

Documentation and handover

- Document risk assessment clearly in maternal healthcare record
- Ensure thorough face-to-face verbal handover between midwives and document (including identified risks) using appropriate structured handover tool
- Repeat risk assessment at handover of care from each midwifery shift and document any supplementary risks identified

FIRST STAGE OF LABOUR

Observations and assessment during first stage

- As a minimum, perform and document the following on partogram at frequencies indicated, unless other clinical reasons to document more frequently:
- temperature: 4-hrly
- blood pressure: 4-hrly
- maternal pulse: hourly

- abdominal palpation followed by vaginal assessment: 4-hrly
- frequency of contractions
- frequency of bladder emptying (test and measure amount voided)
- If not EFM, auscultate fetal heart rate for at least one full minute every 15 min following a contraction
- If FHR abnormality suspected, palpate maternal pulse to differentiate – see **Electronic fetal monitoring** guideline
- Once in established labour, complete partogram

> **Carry out continuous risk assessment to determine whether to transfer to high-risk labour care**

Woman's comfort

- Midwife must also consider:
- regular assessment of woman's emotional and physical state
- ongoing discussion regarding pain relief

Diet and fluids

- Throughout first stage of established labour offer a light, easily digestible diet and encourage fluid intake
- If clinical evidence of dehydration, give IV fluids, either 1 L sodium chloride 0.9% or compound sodium lactate (Hartmann's) solution IV (according to local practice)
- **High-risk women** – clear fluid only

H$_2$ receptor antagonists (antacids)

- **Low-risk women** – not routinely offered (unless opioid analgesia used in labour)
- **High risk women** – offer ranitidine 150 mg oral 6-hrly (if oral inappropriate, 50 mg IM 6-hrly)

Position and mobility

- An upright position during labour facilitates efficient uterine contractions, shortens latent phase and reduces need for analgesia

- Encourage mobilisation
- Allow woman to adopt a position she is comfortable with

Delay in first stage of labour

- See **Delay in labour** guideline

SECOND STAGE OF LABOUR

> **Risk to mother and fetus increases during second stage of labour**

Presumptive diagnosis of second stage

- Overwhelming urge to push
- Presenting part becomes visible
- Woman wants to empty bowels and has heavy mucoid show

Definitive diagnosis

- Full dilatation of cervix on vaginal examination

Maternal observations

- Monitor and record on partogram:
- Temperature: 4-hrly (unless clinical indications for more frequently)
- blood pressure: hourly (unless other indications e.g. medical reasons, epidural *in situ*)
- pulse: hourly (rising pulse rate can signify maternal complication)
- vaginal assessment hourly in active second stage (after abdominal assessment and assessment of vaginal loss)
- frequency and length of contractions: 30 min intervals
- Encourage woman to void bladder and test each void for ketones and protein
- Document fluids given

Fetal observations

Carry out continuous risk assessment to see if transfer to high-risk labour care necessary

- Unless continuous fetal monitoring, intermittent auscultation of FHR after each contraction for at least one full minute every 5 min
- If fetal bradycardia suspected, palpate maternal pulse rate
- Record FHR on partogram (even if using continuous monitoring)
- Note colour of any liquor draining
- Palpate fetal position and abdominal descent of fetal pole
- Document all findings

Care and positioning during second stage

- Provide emotional and psychological support
- Respect woman's choice of position but discourage from lying supine or semi-supine

Delay in second stage/fetal distress

- If delay in second stage suspected, see **Delay in labour** guideline

Preparation for delivery

- Prepare environment and equipment

THIRD STAGE LABOUR

- See **Third stage of labour** guideline

Issue 3
Issued: April 2015
Expires: April 2017

INTRODUCTION

- Latent phase of labour is a normal process during which dynamic physiological and emotional changes (unique to each woman) occur. It is vital that healthcare professionals caring for women in the latent phase of labour appreciate this physical and psychological process

- This guideline is applicable to women expecting a vaginal birth between 37 and 42 weeks' gestation

DEFINITION

- Onset of short, mild, irregular contractions that soften, efface and begin to dilate the cervix from 0–4 cm. Average duration is poorly understood

ANTENATAL ADVICE

- Midwife will discuss process of latent phase of labour with woman in antenatal period before 37 weeks' gestation, providing her with a realistic understanding of what to expect

- Include this topic in parent education classes and, if available locally, provide woman with an information leaflet

- Provide woman and her birth partner(s) with information about the type of support available during the latent phase of labour

- When developing birth plan, discuss coping strategies, as anxiety can impact on the effectiveness of other relaxation techniques

MANAGEMENT

Telephone assessment

- Most women who feel they are in labour make their first contact with midwife by telephone, in order to seek help and advice. This first contact is an important initial assessment, and it is preferable for a midwife to speak directly with the woman

- if contact is from woman's support person, advise him/her that it would be more appropriate for midwife to speak to the woman directly

- In order that advice and reassurance can be based on individual need, obtain a detailed history

- Document discussions, information and advice given

- Retain a record for future reference if woman makes contact again regarding her labour

- Midwife must exercise professional judgement when diagnosing latent phase of labour

Action

- If appropriate, encourage woman to stay at home and continue normal daily activities, light diet and plenty of fluids, ideally with company but to make further contact if her needs change or she requires midwife support

- Advise about pain relief strategies (see below)

- On the third telephone assessment made by a midwife, arrange for woman to attend maternity unit for full maternal and fetal assessment and plan of care

> **After three telephone assessments, midwife must see woman**

Assessment on admission

- See **Labour management** guideline

Vaginal examination

- Following discussion with woman, consider need for vaginal examination

- if, after examination, it is decided woman is not in active labour, encourage her to go home with advice about when and who to contact

Prolonged latency

- If woman readmitted for a third time, and still not in established labour, consider electronic fetal monitoring and repeat assessment

- Advise woman to inform midwife if:

- intensity and frequency of contractions increases

- any change in fetal activity

- vaginal loss

- any other concerns, whether at home or within maternity unit

- If woman unable or reluctant to go home for whatever reason, or requires pain relief and support, care for her in a non-intrusive environment with access to food and drink

- Women remaining in hospital but not deemed to be in established labour require fetal and maternal assessment, depending on risk assessment

- Women in the latent phase of labour should eat and drink as their appetite dictates. Fasting can lead to dehydration and ketosis, resulting in the need for intervention

Pain relief in latent phase

- Relaxation techniques including breathing methods, massage, heat therapy e.g. with wheat bags or hot water bottle, hydrotherapy, aromatherapy and effective support from birth partner

- Hydrotherapy – consider upright positions using a shower as a more effective alternative to soaking in the bath. However if woman becomes tired, soaking in a bath may provide some relief

- Paracetamol 1 g up to 4 g in 24 hr

- TENS machine

- Consider giving pethidine as a last resort, prescribed by a medical practitioner

> ***Women who have been given pethidine during the latent phase should not go home for at least 6–8 hr after administration***

DEFINITIONS

Definition of nationally reportable maternal deaths

Death while pregnant or within one year of end of pregnancy, childbirth or abortion from any cause related to or aggravated by the pregnancy or its management, but not from accidental or incidental causes

Direct

Resulting from obstetric complications of the pregnant state (pregnancy, labour, and puerperium) from interventions, omissions, incorrect treatment or chain of events resulting from any of the above

Indirect

Resulting from previous existing disease or disease that develops during pregnancy not due to direct obstetric causes, but aggravated by the physiological effects of pregnancy

Late death

Occurring between 42 days and one year after abortion, miscarriage or delivery owing to direct or indirect maternal causes

Coincidental death

Occurring from unrelated causes that occur in the pregnancy or puerperium, e.g. road traffic accident

Legal requirements

It is a statutory requirement that healthcare professionals provide information and participate in confidential enquiries. Head of midwifery must ensure other areas of the Trust e.g. A&E, ICU are aware of this requirement

DIRECT MATERNAL DEATH WHILE UNDER MATERNITY CARE

Immediate action

Senior midwife in charge of shift

- Will allocate a member of staff to act as support and will inform:
- head of midwifery
- on-call midwifery manager
- supervisor of midwives
- bereavement officer (where available) as soon as possible within working hours
- on-call consultant
- mortuary

On-call consultant

- Will meet and support relatives
- If cause of death known, request permission for post–mortem
- If cause of death unknown, inform coroner who will order a post-mortem, if he/she feels necessary
- Issue death certificate
- Inform woman's consultant and transfer responsibility for the case if appropriate
- Ensure relatives meet with named obstetric consultant

Midwife in charge of the case

- Will offer support to family
- Document events and secure maternal healthcare record
- Forward photocopy of documents to head of midwifery (original documents may have to go to coroner)
- Participate in review of records
- Inform GP
- Inform named community midwife
- If death occurs outside own area boundaries, notify senior midwife in area woman is booked
- Report as Strategic Executive Information System (STEIS) incident
- Complete local Trust checklist

Member of staff supporting relatives

- Will provide 'What should I do now?' booklet (if available locally)
- Liaise with hospital bereavement officer to arrange religious/spiritual support and completion and issuing of death certificate
- Ensure adequate provision made for baby: consider social services for help and advice particularly if parents not married

Bereavement officer (where available)

- Will be the point of contact for family and medical and midwifery staff
- Offer expert advice and support

Head of midwifery

- Will act as co-ordinator
- Maintain confidential and accurate record of each stage of procedure
- Retain information to feed into current national process
- Work closely with supervisor of midwives
- Provide report detailing events and cause of death to departmental clinical managers, divisional clinical governance manager and Trust chief executive

Supervisor of midwives

- Will notify local supervising authority (LSA) officer using appropriate form
- Review maternal healthcare record with midwife in charge of case and complete a summary. Note names of all staff involved, particularly those who do not normally work within the maternity department e.g. resuscitation team, operating department practitioners

Through the risk management process, identify and arrange support for all staff concerned

MATERNAL DEATH (NOT IN MATERNITY UNIT)

- In the event of a maternal death in hospital but not in the maternity unit, department concerned must notify head of midwifery as soon as possible within normal working hours
- A designated supervisor of midwives will inform LSA officer
- It is the responsibility of the department in which the maternal death occurred to inform coroner's office (where necessary) and to ensure multidisciplinary decision-making in the management of maternal death and level of investigation required (e.g. post-mortem) is documented
- In the case of a death occurring within A&E this is an automatic requirement

DEATH IN PRIMARY CARE

Indirect, coincidental and late

- Deaths in primary care setting may include, murder, suicide, road traffic accident, women with known terminal illness and should be dealt with on an individual basis
- Woman's midwife is responsible for ensuring supervisor of midwives is informed of any maternal death in the primary care setting that comes to her attention
- Supervisor of midwives will inform head of midwifery and LSA
- GP should notify the hospital where woman had delivered or received care
- If maternal death occurs in the community, GP must notify director of public health

Issue 3
Issued: April 2015
Expires: April 2017

BACKGROUND

- Safe transfer or retrieval of a woman from one clinical care setting to another to provide care in specialist area or centre
- Transfers may be made for maternal or neonatal reasons and can occur at any stage of antenatal, intrapartum or postnatal period
- It may be necessary to transfer between community and hospital or from one hospital to another (e.g. where specific maternal/neonatal facilities are required)

This guideline covers

- Transfer into hospital from community
- Transfer to another specialist unit within Trust
- Transfer to maternity unit from within Trust
- Transfer to another Trust
- In-utero transfer
- Postnatal transfer

PREPARATION FOR ALL TRANSFERS

- Before transfer, perform risk assessment and complete local handover tool (e.g. ACCEPT, SBAR)
- Inform clinical staff and woman of reason for transfer
- Document events leading up to decision to transfer, together with a provisional diagnosis
- Before transfer, provide receiving unit with written and verbal summary of woman's condition and provisional diagnosis
- Woman and baby's medical record must accompany them when they transfer
- There should be local agreements with the ambulance service regarding attendance at emergencies or when transfer required
- Urgency of transfer will determine personnel required and mode of transport
- Midwife allocated to woman should monitor fetal wellbeing if applicable

Equipment

- Ensure accompanying equipment functioning with charged batteries
- Supply sufficient drugs and fluids for entire journey
- Secure lines (e.g. IV, CVP, urinary catheter)

Woman

- Explain reason for transfer to woman and partner and document discussion in healthcare record
- Obtain and record consent (where able)
- Stabilise woman for transfer

Fetus

- Assess fetal wellbeing if appropriate

Documentation (requirements for each staff group)

Midwife

- Documentation and handover responsibility, to include:
- summary of maternal transfer documented in woman's healthcare record and continue to complete appropriate tool (e.g. ACCEPT) for handover
- ensure full photo-copy of maternal healthcare record (including EFM traces, drug charts, investigation results etc) accompany woman. If results not available at time of transfer, telephone as soon as available

Medical staff

- If transferring to another hospital, middle grade obstetrician (ST3–7 or equivalent e.g. staff grade, clinical fellow) to write detailed letter containing patient history, sequence of events and treatment, including:
- drugs prescribed and administered
- investigation reports/results
- description of fetal heart rate (FHR) trace
- anaesthetic chart (if applicable)

Prepare for transportation

Personnel

- Qualified midwife must accompany woman
- Specialist personnel (e.g. anaesthetist, obstetrician) may be required to accompany woman, depending on her condition and current condition of the fetus after assessment by person(s) making decision to transfer

Monitoring during transportation

- Continue appropriate monitoring during ambulance transfer until handover at receiving unit

TRANSFER IN FROM COMMUNITY

- Community midwife will:
- identify need for transfer
- inform team leader of appropriate clinical area (depending on condition necessitating transfer). Outline patient history and current maternal and fetal/baby condition using local risk assessment tool

Booking ambulance

- Community midwife will call 999 and request ambulance with paramedic assistance
- Follow local **Home delivery** guideline

On admission to delivery suite

If admitted to delivery suite (e.g. from home birth)

- Most senior obstetrician present on delivery suite will review within 30 min of admission
- If no immediate concerns, perform initial risk assessment and request middle grade obstetrician (ST3–7 or equivalent e.g. staff grade, clinical fellow) to review as soon as possible
- Wherever appropriate and possible, community midwife responsible for transfer should continue to care for woman

TRANSFER TO OTHER SPECIALIST UNIT WITHIN TRUST

- Daily review by senior obstetrician:
- antenatal/postnatal assessment by delivery suite team leader to ensure antenatal/postnatal care maintained
- document subsequent treatment/ discussions in woman's healthcare record

> *Decision to transfer woman to other specialist unit within Trust (e.g. critical care area) must be made by consultant obstetrician and consultant anaesthetist after discussion with senior staff in receiving area (e.g. intensive care consultant)*

Booking transport

- Midwife will arrange transport (e.g. ambulance or porter) as per local practice

TRANSFER TO MATERNITY UNIT FROM WITHIN TRUST

> *Multidisciplinary decision involving transferring team, receiving team, consultant obstetrician and midwife*

- Midwife in charge will inform all appropriate members of maternity team of impending arrival
- He/she will ensure full handover from transferring department, including:
- history
- healthcare record accompanies woman
- drugs prescribed/administered
- investigation requests/results

TRANSFER FROM DELIVERY SUITE TO ANOTHER TRUST

- Delivery suite on-call consultant obstetrician will make decision to transfer woman
- Once decision confirmed, midwife team leader and middle grade obstetrician (ST3–7 or equivalent e.g. staff grade, clinical fellow) will co-ordinate arrangements and allocate tasks to team members

Issue 3
Issued: April 2015
Expires: April 2017

- If anaesthetic referral required, consultant anaesthetist will contact consultant anaesthetist at receiving unit directly

Booking ambulance

- Person making decision will indicate transportation required. Consultation with neonatologist and anaesthetist may be necessary
- Transfer co-ordinator will allocate the task of booking ambulance to a team member, who will:
- book ambulance, indicating urgency
- request specific equipment (e.g. stretcher, oxygen, portable ventilator)
- indicate number of personnel accompanying woman (dependent upon multidisciplinary team assessment)
- request estimated time of arrival

Arrival at receiving unit

- Escorting staff should:
- handover to receiving team, giving information on vital signs, therapy and significant clinical events during transfer
- handover documents
- document details of transfer process in maternal healthcare record until transfer of care completed

IN-UTERO TRANSFER

- In-utero transfer is a major disruption for women and their families and often carries significant risks. It is essential that the woman and her family are involved in the decision-making process and have given their consent to proceed
- If woman is being transferred antenatally due to lack of neonatal facilities, delivery suite team member must locate a unit able to accept mother and baby before any further arrangements are made
- Consultant obstetrician makes decision for in-utero transfer after robust risk assessment discussion with midwife and neonatologist

Indications for in-utero transfer out

- Suspected or actual preterm labour <34 weeks' gestation when no neonatal intensive care unit (NICU) cot available
- Women <34 weeks' gestation requiring delivery for fetal or maternal reasons when no NICU cot available
- Unit unable to safely facilitate management of high-risk cases due to delivery suite activity
- Specialist neonatal care not available at local unit e.g. elective early postnatal surgery indicated for neonate

Indications not to transfer out

- Where transfer may pose a significant risk to mother or baby, continue management locally and instigate ex-utero transfer as necessary e.g:
- advanced labour
- pathological EFM
- unstable mother
- This list is not exhaustive

Procedure

- Ensure careful risk assessment of maternal and fetal condition throughout the transfer process, looking for any deterioration in maternal/fetal wellbeing. Follow your local Trust in-utero transfer guideline
- It is good practice to ensure woman receives appropriate follow-up

POSTNATAL TRANSFER

- If transferring woman alone postnatally, midwife will discharge baby to the care of woman's partner/relatives
- If unable to discharge baby to family, arrange care on postnatal ward

FOLLOWING SAFE TRANSFER OR RETRIEVAL OF WOMAN

- Complete and file all local handover tools in maternal healthcare record
- Delivery suite team leader reports/ documents transfer of woman as per local practice

BACKGROUND

- Meconium stained liquor occurs in 10–20% of deliveries, increasing to over 30% after 42 weeks' gestation

- Meconium aspiration syndrome occurs in 2–5% of babies born through meconium stained liquor

- Significant meconium at onset of labour carries the worst prognosis and is associated with five or seven-fold increased risk of perinatal death

DEFINITION

Significant

- Dark green or black amniotic fluid that is thick or tenacious or any meconium stained amniotic fluid containing lumps of meconium

Light

- Staining of lesser severity

MANAGEMENT

- Unless birth imminent, transfer from low-risk setting to care of an obstetrician

- If woman is not in labour and thick meconium is present, arrange induction of labour

- Continuous electronic fetal monitoring (EFM) is advised for women with significant meconium stained liquor – see **Electronic fetal monitoring** guideline

In labour

- Whatever the degree or time of passage of meconium, fetal risks are increased

- If fetal heart rate abnormalities also present, perform fetal blood sampling – see **Fetal blood sampling** guideline

- When delivery imminent, call neonatal team according to local practice

- Take umbilical cord sample – see **Umbilical cord sampling** guideline

- Report meconium change from light to significant to middle grade obstetrician (ST3–7 or equivalent e.g. staff grade, clinical fellow)

RESUSCITATION OF BABIES BORN FROM MECONIUM STAINED LIQUOR

Ensure resuscitation equipment is checked and ready for use before delivery

Active baby

- If baby crying and active at birth:
  - dry and cover to avoid hypothermia
  - **do not** aspirate airways
  - neonatologist **does not** inspect larynx or aspirate trachea (unnecessary intubation and lower airway suction does more harm than good)

Floppy baby

- If baby floppy, pale and makes no immediate respiratory effort at birth, call neonatal team (if not already present) and commence neonatal resuscitation – see **Cardiopulmonary resuscitation of the newborn** guideline (**Airway**) or follow local guidance

- Obtain arterial and venous cord blood to asses pH and blood gases – see **Umbilical cord sampling** guideline and record values in maternal healthcare record and, if local practice, in neonatal notes

Postnatal observations

- For any baby delivered with a history of significant meconium, perform the following observations at 1 and 2 hr of age and then 2-hrly until 12 hr of age. Document in neonatal observations chart:
  - general wellbeing
  - chest movement and nasal flare
  - skin colour including perfusion by capillary refill
  - feeding
  - muscle tone
  - temperature
  - heart rate and respiration
- If light meconium staining occurred, observations for baby as above at 1 and 2 hr of age and document in neonatal observations chart
- If baby's condition causes concern at any time, review by neonatologist

Issue 3
Issued: April 2015
Expires: April 2017

INTRODUCTION

- Obtain written informed consent, together with written agreement of two certified medical practitioners who have signed HSA1 form (Abortion act 1967 revised 1991)

- Guidance from Royal College of Obstetricians and Gynaecologists on termination of pregnancy for fetal abnormality stresses that a legal abortion 'must not be allowed to result in a live birth' www.rcog.org.uk/search/node/termination. Therefore, method of termination of pregnancy after 21 weeks, should ensure fetus is born dead

- Where termination is planned >21+6 weeks for abnormalities that are not lethal, consultant in fetal medicine must discuss fetocide with woman

- If woman refuses fetocide, document clearly in notes that it has been offered and declined

RECOMMENDED DRUG REGIMEN

Initial drug dose

- Mifepristone (Mifegyne RU 486) 200 mg oral is administered by senior obstetrician on licensed premises and a healthcare professional must observe woman take tablet

- Inform woman of possibility of abdominal discomfort and/or a small amount of bleeding

- reassure that this is normal and can be treated with regular paracetamol at home

- Ask woman to remain on premises for 1 hour to observe side effects

- if vomiting occurs, repeat dose

- Induction may commence at this point or, should the woman wish, she may go home and return the following day

- Provide contact telephone numbers with instructions to call if she has any concerns while at home. If available locally, give patient information leaflet

Further drug regimen

- No more than 24–72 hr after initial dose of mifepristone 200 mg oral, give misoprostol:

- **<26 week's gestation:** 100 microgram vaginally 6-hrly – **maximum 4 doses**

- **>27 week's gestation:** 25–50 microgram vaginally 4-hrly – **maximum 6 doses**

> *In previous caesarean section or uterine surgery, where the cavity has been breached (e.g. myomectomy, uterine perforation) use 25–50 microgram dosage*

Side effects/complications associated with misoprostol

- Pyrexia
- Diarrhoea
- Retained placenta
- Hypovolaemic shock
- Ruptured uterus
- Extra vigilance in women with:
- severe asthma
- previous operative delivery
- cardiovascular insufficiency
- previous caesarean section
- anticoagulant treatment
- renal/hepatic failure
- long-term corticosteroid therapy
- Advise woman she may experience flu like symptoms e.g. feeling feverish or rise in temperature

INTRAPARTUM MANAGEMENT

- See **Fetal loss** guideline

Management of third stage

- Actively manage according to **Third stage of labour** guideline

- In general, woman should be cared for as if she had experienced any other fetal loss (see **Fetal loss** guideline)

Notifying Department of Health

- Doctor responsible for commencing termination of pregnancy is required, by law, to notify Department of Health by submitting relevant (yellow HSA4) form

FETOCIDE

If not performed locally, refer to regional centre

Definition

- Intracardiac injection of potassium chloride to induce fetal death before termination of pregnancy

Informed consent

- Counsel woman about reasons for carrying out fetocide and explain legal position and ethical implications should baby be born alive

Pre-termination assessment

- Carried out by trained staff who will provide counselling and support

- Perform ultrasound scan immediately before procedure to confirm presence of fetal abnormalities and select suitable site for needle entry

- For fetus with chromosomal abnormality, scan features may not be present. Laboratory report must be available to consultant before fetocide performed

Procedure

- Identify suitable entry site and clean abdomen and probe with antiseptic solution

- Anaesthetise skin and subcutaneous tissues with lidocaine 1% 5–10 mL

- Draw 1.5 g (10 mL potassium chloride 15% KCl) into a new syringe

- Place sterile aqueous gel onto probe to facilitate scanning

- Under ultrasound guidance, insert 21 gauge echo tip needle into fetal heart

- Using a 5 mL syringe, withdraw a small volume of fetal blood to confirm correct placement of needle. If required, send blood for cytogenetic analysis

- Slowly inject 5–8 mL KCl solution into fetal heart until cardiac activity stops

- Allow mother to rest for 5–10 min before performing a confirmatory scan to check fetal cardiac activity has not resumed

- Transfer mother to delivery suite to complete termination

DEFINITION

- Placenta adheres to or invades the myometrium

Increased incidence

- If placenta is located over a previous scar
- With increasing number of caesarean sections
- Following myomectomy
- If previous manual removal of placenta from the same placental site

> **Morbidly adherent placenta carries an increased risk of mortality due to massive obstetric haemorrhage at delivery**

ANTENATAL CARE

- Advise ultrasound scan at 20 weeks' gestation to determine placental site
- if scan reveals a low or anterior placenta with a history of previous caesarean section, further ultrasound scan at 32 weeks' gestation to identify distance from lower edge of the placenta to cervical os and determine whether the placenta overlies the old scar
- report signs of invasion of the scar by placental tissue
- a colour-flow Doppler ultrasound scan performed by an experienced sonographer is the first line diagnostic test
- Where the placenta lies over the old scar, or in placenta praevia, consultant obstetrician will discuss with woman (and her partner if appropriate) and plan antenatal care including further imaging and multi-disciplinary preparation and delivery
- MRI scan, arranged with a consultant radiologist, can aid diagnosis and clarify depth of invasion
- Since up to 40% of cases are likely to require emergency delivery, place a clear care plan in woman's healthcare record and hand-held notes
- Discuss the risk of hysterectomy

- Re-check haemoglobin after 32 weeks' gestation and, if anaemic, prescribe oral iron
- Refer woman to an obstetric anaesthetist

Advice to woman

- If appropriate, inform woman and her partner about the risk of major haemorrhage and advise to:
- avoid sexual intercourse for the remainder of the pregnancy
- contact maternity triage to attend hospital immediately if any vaginal blood loss, contractions, pain or suprapubic period-like aches
- ensure someone available at home who can help and take to hospital if necessary

ELECTIVE DELIVERY

- Schedule elective caesarean section at 36–37 weeks' gestation
- Give antenatal steroids to reduce risk of respiratory distress syndrome
- Multidisciplinary planning involving consultant obstetrician, consultant anaesthetist and haematologist
- Ensure 4–6 units of packed red blood cells available in delivery suite blood fridge on morning of procedure and a senior haematologist available for advice
- An experienced neonatologist to be present at birth
- A scan on morning of procedure may be useful in mapping placental site
- Arrange a perfusionist to facilitate cell salvage if required
- Where there is high probability of a morbidly adherent placenta it may be appropriate to liaise with an interventional radiologist if available locally
- it may be appropriate to insert balloons in the femoral arteries before procedure as a prophylactic measure for inflation in the event of postpartum haemorrhage. Particularly appropriate for women who will not consent to a blood transfusion
- Ensure local availability of level 2 critical care bed

Consent

● Must be taken by a consultant obstetrician who will discuss blood transfusion, hysterectomy, admission to critical care and the possibility of leaving the placenta in place. It will include routine consent for caesarean section

● If placenta left *in situ* – pregnancies have been reported after this approach but so have cases of delayed haemorrhage and hysterectomy

Procedure

● Consultant obstetric anaesthetist will determine and administer type of anaesthetic

● Consultant obstetrician must perform caesarean section

● It may be appropriate to open the lower segment of the uterus, thus leaving a lower segment scar only. However, it may be appropriate to access the uterine cavity deliberately avoiding the placenta. This requires knowledge of the limits of the placental site. This approach allows an assessment of placental adherence without heavy bleeding before a definitive decision is made

● If the placenta separates, the operation continues as normal

● If it remains adherent, there are two options:

  ○ proceed directly to hysterectomy or

  ○ leave the placenta *in situ* and manage conservatively in the postnatal period

● Even if placenta is thought to be morbidly adherent and not bleeding at time of caesarean section, give 5 units of Syntocinon IV slowly to ensure placenta does not separate and is truly adherent

● If placenta is clearly adherent, do not continue to remove it

● If plan of care is to manage the placenta *in situ* conservatively, unclamp the cord and drain the placenta of blood before tying off and dividing the cord as close to its insertion into the placenta as surgically practicable

● Close the uterus in the routine way or proceed directly to hysterectomy

● If the placenta separates, partially adherent portion(s) can be left in place. Heavy blood loss can occur – see **Postpartum haemorrhage** guideline

Postnatal care

● Provide level 2 critical care for at least 2 hr after delivery

● Regularly assess uterine fundus and observe carefully for signs of haemorrhage. Where a placenta totally covering the cervical os is left *in situ*, it can conceal bleeding within the uterine cavity. In this situation, woman should remain on delivery suite for 24 hr

Management when placenta left *in situ* postnatally

● Carries risk of infection and delayed haemorrhage. Ensure woman understands the need for a commitment to hospital visits for clinical checks, blood tests and possibly imaging

● Antibiotic prophylaxis can be used a few days after delivery but postnatal follow-up with prompt recognition and treatment of any infection is more important. This requires twice-weekly hospital visits with clinical review, blood tests for FBC and C reactive protein

● Monitor placental re-absorption weekly with serum Beta hCG levels and ultrasound. There have been reports of methotrexate use and of elective ERPC at 6 weeks postnatally

RISKS

- Perinatal mortality (six times higher)
- Small for gestational age
- Congenital malformation
- Cerebral palsy (four times higher)
- Birth asphyxia higher for second twin, usually occurs after delivery of first twin
- Twin-to-twin transfusion in monozygotic twins
- Cord entanglement and locking in monochorionic monoamniotic twins
- Preterm labour
- Maternal morbidity higher:
- anaemia
- placenta praevia
- pre-eclampsia
- postpartum haemorrhage

ANTENATAL MANAGEMENT

- Follow local antenatal care pathway
- If multiple pregnancy suspected, ultrasound scan to confirm and ensure woman under consultant care
- In twin pregnancy ultrasonographer will determine chorionicity in the first trimester. Chorionicity determines the degree of risk and management
- If a woman wishes to have pre-labour caesarean section, administer antenatal steroids for fetal lung maturity

Communication

- Discuss plan of care with parents, ensuring sufficient information given
- Provide psychological support and, where possible, written information and contact details of multiple pregnancy support groups

Plan of care (in addition to routine antenatal care)

- Undertake FBC at 20–24 weeks' gestation and have low threshold for iron and folic acid supplementation

- Offer first trimester combined Down's syndrome screening
- Second trimester serum screening not appropriate in multiple pregnancy
- At each antenatal examination after 24 weeks' gestation, confirm presence of two fetal hearts using Pinnards, sonic aid or ultrasound scan
- **Monochorionic pregnancy between 16–24 weeks' gestation:**
- scan every 2 weeks, looking for twin-to-twin transfusion syndrome (TTS)
- if TTS suspected, refer to local fetal medicine consultant
- **Dichorionic pregnancy and monochorionic pregnancy after 24 weeks:**
- perform serial growth scan at least every 4 weeks
- 20 week detailed scan to detect fetal anomalies
- If growth of one of the fetuses falls below projected centile, ask consultant obstetrician to plan further management
- In the event of death of one twin, discuss with fetal medicine consultant

Delivery plan

Twins

- Detailed counselling by senior obstetrician regarding mode, place and timing of delivery
- Monochorionic dichorionic pregnancy: offer delivery at 36 weeks
- Dichorionic pregnancy: offer delivery at 37 weeks
- Monochorionic monoamniotic pregnancy: offer caesarean section at 32 weeks

Triplets and higher order pregnancies

- Must be delivered in a unit with sufficient and appropriate neonatal intensive care (NICU) facilities

INTRAPARTUM MANAGEMENT (TWIN PREGNANCY)

First stage of labour

- On admission, inform middle grade obstetrician (ST3–7 or equivalent e.g. staff grade, clinical fellow) and consultant

- Confirm presence of two fetal hearts using Pinnards or sonic aid

- if two separate fetal hearts difficult to identify, ultrasound scan

- Unless contraindicated because of extreme prematurity, continuous electronic monitoring of fetal hearts

- if difficulty monitoring two separate fetal hearts at any time, consider fetal scalp electrode or ultrasound scan

> *Inability to continuously monitor both babies despite use of ultrasound scan to ascertain placement of transducers and a fetal scalp electrode if appropriate, is an indication for caesarean section*

- Insert IV cannula and flush

- Take blood for full blood count (FBC) and group and save

- Review obstetric records, fetal presentation and plan for delivery

- discuss plan of care with parents and document in maternal healthcare record

- While respecting woman's choice, encourage her to use epidural analgesia to facilitate delivery in the event of internal manoeuvres or urgent instrumental delivery becoming necessary

- If oxytocin required to accelerate labour [prescribed by middle grade obstetrician (ST3–7 or equivalent e.g. staff grade, clinical fellow) or consultant only], use with caution

Second stage of labour

Ensure

- Experienced obstetric consultant, middle grade obstetrician (ST3–7 or equivalent e.g. staff grade, clinical fellow), neonatology team and midwives are present in room at delivery

- Appropriate equipment, including:
  - ultrasound machine
  - resuscitation equipment

- Anaesthetist and theatre team on standby on labour ward

- In the case of caesarean section, one midwife per baby is designated to receive the babies

- Oxytocin as per local practice

- If all normal, midwife will carry out delivery, otherwise middle grade obstetrician (ST3–7 or equivalent e.g. staff grade, clinical fellow) or consultant will perform

- Deliver twin one and place one clamp on umbilical cord

Delivery of second twin

- **Aim to deliver second twin within 30 min**

- risk for second twin increases steeply as time passes from delivery of first twin

- Continuous electronic fetal monitoring

- Determine presentation and lie

- Monitor vaginal loss

- Perform abdominal palpation to determine presentation. At the same time, perform a vaginal examination – preferably by middle grade obstetrician (ST3–7 or equivalent e.g. staff grade, clinical fellow) or consultant to allow interventions, if appropriate, without repeat examination

- where second twin was not cephalic in first stage of labour, it may be appropriate to deliver the woman in lithotomy to allow rapid vaginal examination of second twin and perform interventions as required

Issue 3
Issued: April 2015
Expires: April 2017

- Stabilise second twin as longitudinal lie

- Prepare ultrasound machine in case required to confirm position of second twin

- If necessary, perform external cephalic version

- Where second twin was not cephalic in first stage of labour it may be appropriate to deliver the woman in lithotomy to allow rapid vaginal examination of second twin and perform interventions as required

- internal podalic version and breech extraction before cervix can shrink

- If any delay in resumption of effective uterine contractions, start oxytocin infusion according to local practice at maximum rate

- If vertex or breech in pelvis, perform artificial rupture of membranes at peak of contraction

- After delivery of second twin, place two clamps on umbilical cord

Active management of third stage of labour

- Oxytocin infusion as per local practice

- Cord gases

- Because of risk of haemorrhage, avoid too rapid transfer to postnatal ward

INTRODUCTION

This guideline provides a framework for management of neuropraxias after central neuroaxial blockade (CNB) e.g. spinal or epidural. Incidence: (1:2,000). The peripheral nerve, lumbosacral plexus and conus medularis can be damaged by maternal posture or fetal head pressure directly on nerves or nutrient blood vessels

Before administering regional anaesthesia, provide woman with information on potential neurological complications

PREVENTING NEUROLOGICAL DAMAGE

- Chlorhexidine is the skin preparation of choice. Allow to dry completely

- **Do not** splash chlorhexidine on spinal or epidural needles

- If, on performing CNB, there are recurrent, persistent, bilateral or severe symptoms of dysaesthesia, reconsider further attempts

- To maintain spinal cord perfusion, prevent prolonged periods of hypotensive episodes

- Follow local guidance for regional blocks and regional anaesthesia for the anticoagulated woman

- Avoid neuroaxial procedures in the septic patient (discuss with on-call consultant) or in the presence of localised infection

- When topping up with heavy concentration of local anaesthetic, ensure proper surgical positioning

> *Redosing of subarachnoid local anaesthetic, beyond recommended doses may increase the risk of spinal cord neurotoxicity*

Risk factors for neurological deficits

Pre-existing neurological disorders (e.g. multiple sclerosis, diabetes mellitus, extremes of body habitus, direct trauma, stretch, improper patient positioning)

TYPES OF NEUROLOGICAL DEFICITS

- Short-lived nerve damage occurs around 1:300 after an obstetric CNB and permanent neuropathy occurs in about 1:15,000

- Peripheral nerve injuries (1:2000)

- Neurotoxicity

- Mechanical (direct needle or catheter)

- Arachnoiditis

- Ischaemic injury

- Disc herniation (1:10,000)

- Meningitis (1:100,000)

- Central compressive neuropathy (haematoma 1:168,000)

- Abscess 1:145,000

RECOGNITION OF NEUROLOGICAL DEFICIT

- Early detection is critical in managing spinal cord ischaemia, vertebral canal haematoma and abscess. After 8 hr, the likelihood of full or partial recovery rapidly diminishes

- Some recovery of motor blockade must be seen within 4 hr of CNB

- If dense block still present, anaesthetist to perform baseline neurological assessment

- Institute half-hourly leg muscle strength monitoring alongside routine hourly monitoring and record on MEWS score chart

Dense block after regional analgesia

- If abnormal block develops on routine epidural analgesia regimen, stop infusion immediately

- If a denser blockade develops, involve senior anaesthetist urgently

- If not recovered in 4 hr, consider prompt MRI scan

- If recovery occurs, restart epidural infusion but maintain neurological surveillance

- If block recurs, abandon epidural and investigate

- Continue neurological assessment in HDU for 24 hr
- If haematoma suspected, do not remove catheter

Subdural block can cause a dense, very persistent block that is frequently unilateral

Neurological impairment after CNB

See flowchart for Management of neurological impairment after CNB

Review woman

- Presentation will vary with the aetiology
- Nerve damage by epidural and spinal needles is associated with paraesthesia (1:3,000)

Epidural haematoma

- Leg weakness and sensory symptoms are more common than back pain. They usually progress rapidly and may be unilateral

Meningitis

- Meningitis after dural puncture usually presents with severe headache. Onset of nuchal rigidity, photophobia, confusion and pyrexia may be delayed

Infective meningitis suspected

- Consult neurologist and microbiologist urgently
- If pyrexial, send blood cultures
- If epidural infection suspected. send epidural catheter tip and swab of entry site for MS+S
- Early diagnostic lumbar puncture

Disc herniation

- Presents as severe back pain, bilateral sciatica and motor weakness in the legs
- Cauda equina compression due to centrally prolapsed discs presents as saddle anaesthesia, urinary retention and reduced anal tone

Red flag signs

- Unexpected dense motor block
- Markedly increasing motor block, including unilateral block, motor block that does not recede and recurrent motor blockade
- Severe or worsening backache
- Bowel and bladder dysfunction
- Radicular pain

MANAGEMENT OF NEUROLOGICAL INVOLVEMENT

Testing for neurological involvement

- Test myotomes, dermatomes and reflexes

URGENT (space occupying lesions suspected)

Complete or progressive neurological deficits

- Urgent evaluation by spinal surgeon
- Urgent MRI scan

Lesions with moderate to severe deficits

- Require a more urgent referral to either a spinal surgeon or neurologist
- Consider MRI scan

NOT URGENT

Mild or resolving symptoms

- Without objective evidence of neural deficit typically indicates excellent prognosis requiring reassurance only
- If no improvement in 4–6 weeks, seek neurological advice and refer to neurologist
- Neurophysiological investigation
- After initial evaluation, follow up incomplete and unresolved injuries in 3–6 months

Infective meningitis suspected

- Consult neurologist
- Early diagnostic lumbar puncture and antibiotics

Investigations for neuroaxial injury

- For suspected lesions, MRI scan is the diagnostic investigation of choice
- If MRI scan not immediately available, use CT scan for rapid diagnosis of compressive injuries

Neurophysiological studies

- Together with an MRI scan, can help quantify and locate injury site
- Neurophysiological changes are most apparent after 14–21 days of injury
- Earlier testing may be indicated to rule out pre-existing disease, establish baseline and aid prognosis

Management of a neurological deficit after CNB

Neurological deficit identified

↓

History:	Emphasis on labour, drugs and neurology
Examination:	Neurological and back examination
Anaesthetic:	Review technique

↓

Clinical diagnosis suggestive of

↓

Spinal epidural space occupying lesion

- Urgent consultant review
- Urgent MRI scan
- Liaise with spinal surgeon
- Contract obstetrician

Suspected peripheral nerve damage

If motor block present
- Urgent MRI scan and nerve conduction studies
- Refer to physiotherapist
- Follow-up in 6–12 weeks

No evidence of neurological deficit

- Reassure woman
- Arrange next day follow-up
- Document findings

If being discharged, warn about acute onset back ache, radicular pain, lower extremity weakness and numbness, urinary and anal dysfunction

Issue 3
Issued: April 2015
Expires: April 2017

Leg weakness with epidural analgesia – Management flowchart for midwife

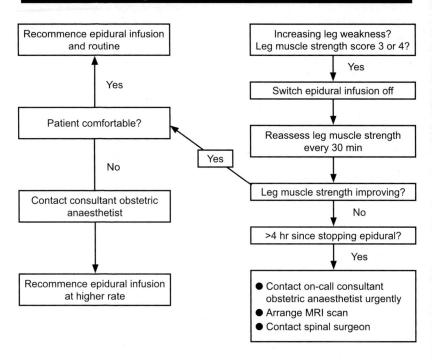

Laboratory test	Value
Hb	110–140 g/L
WCC	6–16 x 10^9/L
Platelets	150–400 x 10^9/L
MCV	80–100 fl
CRP	0–7 g/L
Sodium	130–140 mmol/L
Potassium	3.3–4.1 mmol/L
Urea	<4.5 mmol/L
Creatinine	<75 µmol/L
Urates	<380 µmol/L If 350–380, middle grade/consultant reviews notes
24 hr protein	0.3 g
Protein creatinine ratio	>30 mg/mmol
Creatinine clearance	80–170 mL/min
Bilirubin	≤16 µmol/L
Total protein	48–64 g/L
Albumin	28–37 g/L
AST	10–30 iu/L
ALT	6–32 iu/L
GGT	3–43 iu/L
Alkaline phosphate	30–418 iu/L
Bile acids	≤14 µmol/L

Issue 3
Issued: April 2015
Expires: April 2017

DEFINITION

● Body mass index (BMI) = weight in kg/height in metres squared (m^2)
● WHO classifies women with BMI >30 as obese

Table 1: Classification of body mass index

Classification	BMI	Risk of co-morbidities
Underweight	<18.5	Low (but increased risk of other clinical problems)
Desirable weight	18.5–24.9	Average
Overweight	25.0–29.9	Mildly increased
Obese	>30.0	
Class I	30.0–34.9	Moderate
Class II	35.0–39.9	High
Class III (severely or morbidly obese)	>40.0	Very high

● Risks associated with pregnancy and childbirth are significant when BMI >35
● In this guideline, obesity will be defined as ≥35 kg/m2 during pregnancy, delivery and postnatal period

RISKS OF OBESITY

Mother			Baby
Pregnancy	**Intrapartum**	**Postnatal**	
● Maternal death or severe morbidity ● Cardiac disease ● Spontaneous first trimester and recurrent miscarriage ● Pre-eclampsia and hypertension ● Thromboembolism ● Gestational diabetes ● Infection e.g. urinary tract infection, genital infection	● Increased risk of difficult fetal monitoring ● Inadequate analgesia ● Increased anaesthetic risks ● Increased need for induction of labour ● Slow progress in labour ● Shoulder dystocia ● Operative delivery ● Increased risk of emergency caesarean section (CS) ● Difficult CS with greater mortality and morbidity	● Thromboembolism ● Increased maternal mortality ● Post CS wound infection ● Infection from other causes ● Postnatal infection ● Postpartum haemorrhage ● Perineal tears ● Low breastfeeding rates	● Congenital abnormalities ● Prematurity ● Stillbirth and neonatal death ● Macrosomia (birth trauma) with associated risk of shoulder dystocia ● Fetal abnormalities including neural tube defect ● Admission to Neonatal Intensive Care Unit (NICU) ● Intrauterine growth restriction (IUGR) ● Obesity (in later life)

Difficulties in maternal treatment

- Moving and handling injuries to woman and staff
- Venepuncture/abdominal examination/blood pressure assessment
- Regional and general anaesthesia
- Monitoring during labour
- Performing ultrasound scans, including risk of failure to detect abnormalities

ENVIRONMENT AND EQUIPMENT

- Adequate doorway widths and thresholds
- Theatre trolley and operating table able to take weight >180 kg
- Examination and ultrasound couch able to take weight >180 kg
- Delivery and ward bed able to take weight >180 kg
- Moving equipment e.g. hover mattress or hoist
- Large chairs without arms
- Large wheelchairs
- Calibrated weighing scale
- Height measuring equipment
- Range of epidural and spinal needles, including extra-long
- Appropriately sized thromboembolic stockings
- Appropriately sized theatre gowns
- Large blood pressure cuffs

MANAGEMENT BEFORE CONCEPTION

- Offer pre-pregnancy counselling on lifestyle, diet and smoking cessation
- encourage women who wish to lose weight to follow a weight reduction programme and take regular exercise at least 2–3 months before pregnancy
- consider referral to dietitian
- consider referral to smoking cessation advisor (if available)

- Screen for diabetes
- High dose folic acid 5 mg/day
- Record blood pressure

> ***Obese women require the same routine antenatal, intrapartum and postnatal care as all other women***

INITIAL ANTENATAL CARE

- Refer for consultant-led care and advise woman to give birth in a consultant-led unit
- if woman requests home birth, inform supervisor of midwives
- Venous thromboembolism (VTE) risk assessment and follow **VTE thromboprophylaxis** guideline
- Early booking visit to antenatal clinic to plan pregnancy

At booking

- Measure height and weight and calculate BMI for all women
- Record arm circumference (to ensure appropriate BP cuff used) in maternal healthcare record, customised growth chart (if used) and computerised maternal system (if used locally)
- note inter-pregnancy weight change
- Blood pressure using large cuff – see **Table**
- Assess venous thromboembolism (VTE) risk
- Anticipate requirement for specific equipment during labour and document in maternal healthcare record

Cuff	Arm circumference range at midpoint (cm)
Adult	27–34
Large adult	35–44
Adult thigh cuff	45–52

Book

- Anomaly scan. Inform ultrasound department of obese woman to ensure correct couch used and longer appointment time
- Glucose tolerance test (GTT) at 26–28 weeks' gestation

Discussion with woman

- Explain significance of BMI to woman. Provide advice on weight management, including lifestyle and diet
- where available, give written information on diet and risk of obesity in pregnancy
- offer referral to dietitian and/or weight management programme
- advise ≥30 min/day moderate physical activity (e.g. walking, swimming, aqua-natal) on 5 or more days per week
- Advice on breastfeeding

Prophylaxis treatment

- Advise vitamin D supplement ('Healthy start' vitamins)
- Severely obese women (BMI >35 kg/m^2) plus one additional risk factor for hypertensive disease, prescribe aspirin 75 mg/day from 12 weeks' gestation

VTE prophylaxis

- If admitted to hospital or other intercurrent problems develop, repeat VTE risk assessment

Referrals

- Based on individual needs refer to:
- dietitian and/or weight management programme accordingly to local protocol
- if BMI >40: anaesthetics (if available locally, give anaesthetics information leaflet)
- for smoking cessation – according to local protocol

Communication

- Complete local alert form
- Discuss with manual handling department to ensure appropriate equipment available
- Inform senior delivery suite midwife to ensure availability of appropriate equipment – see **Environment and equipment** above
- If mobility reduced, seek advice from manual handling department

SUBSEQUENT ANTENATAL CARE

- Routine antenatal care and:
- it may be appropriate to re-weigh woman in third trimester
- serial ultrasound scan for fetal growth
- increased risk of gestational diabetes – book GTT as per local policy
- In third trimester with BMI >40:
- provide information about tissue viability
- manual handling assessment
- Offer continued advice and support. Encourage weight gain to be kept to 7–10 kg

ANAESTHETIC ASSESSMENT AND MANAGEMENT

Assessment

- Consider likelihood of difficult intubation and airway management – see **General anaesthesia and failed intubation** guideline
- Other co-morbidities may impact on anaesthesia:
- hypertension
- ischaemic heart disease
- respiratory distress
- sleep apnoea
- diabetes
- assess difficult IV cannulation and lumbar anatomy
- Assess on individual basis and according to local protocol

Management

- If anaesthetic or airway management problems anticipated, ask anaesthetist to review who will:
- document plan of care clearly in maternal healthcare record
- discuss plan of care with woman

INTRAPARTUM CARE

- Individual plan of care depending on woman's needs
- Review antenatal anaesthetic assessment and obstetric plan
- Tissue viability assessment and manual handling assessment for labour as per local practice
- Notify duty anaesthetist and middle grade obstetrician (ST3–7 or equivalent e.g. staff grade, clinical fellow) of admission
- Cannulate using wide bore cannula (BMI >40)
- Bloods for FBC and group and save (BMI >40)
- Risk assessment for thromboembolism, document and follow plan
- antiemboletic stockings (if local practice)
- Early epidural may be required for regional analgesia

Monitor

- Fetal monitoring – See **Electronic fetal monitoring (EFM)** guideline
- where difficulty monitoring fetal heart with EFM, apply fetal scalp electrode (FSE)
- If uncertainty about fetal presentation, consider ultrasound scan
- Monitor progress in labour closely. Be aware of increased risk of shoulder dystocia and postpartum haemorrhage (BMI >40)

First and second stage of labour

- Keep as mobile as possible
- Maintain hydration
- Antacid (e.g. ranitidine) as per local policy
- Pressure area care
- If instrumental delivery contemplated, consider performing trial in theatre with an experienced obstetrician (following usual discussion of risks and alternatives). Obesity is a recognised predictor of abandoned trial, shoulder dystocia and birth injury

Third stage of labour

- Active management
- Oxytocin infusion over 4 hr following delivery to reduce risk of postpartum haemorrhage
- Care when putting woman in lithotomy to avoid tissue damage

Caesarean section

- If caesarean section considered – seek advice from consultant obstetrician and anaesthetist – see **Caesarean section** guideline
- Due to risk of poor wound healing, especially if BMI >40, use delayed absorbable suture e.g. PDS for rectus sheath closure
- close subcutaneous fat to prevent wound infection and dehiscence
- a redivac drain can be left above sheath, and interrupted sutures can be used for skin
- Use correct equipment for patient handling including theatre table and bed – See **Equipment**

POSTPARTUM CARE

- Document care in maternal healthcare record
- If operative delivery, consider transfer to high dependency area for immediate postnatal care – see **High dependency care** guideline
- Thromboembolism risk assessment immediately after delivery
- thromboprophylaxis – see **VTE – Thromboprophylaxis** guideline
- adequate analgesia to allow early mobilisation
- antiemboletic stockings
- Encourage good hydration
- If intrathecal opiates not used, consider patient controlled analgesia (PCA)
- Obesity carries increased risk of postnatal wound and genital tact infection. Encourage good hygiene and monitor for signs of infection
- If caesarean section carried out, observe for wound infection, wound dehiscence, DVT, PE and chest infection

PLAN FOR DISCHARGE

- Continue to encourage healthy eating and exercise, reinforcing benefits of a healthy BMI for future wellbeing and subsequent pregnancies. Consider dietitian referral
- Consider referral to physiotherapist
- Unless contraindicated, encourage breastfeeding. Obese women have decreased rates of breastfeeding (initiation and maintenance) but it can help with postnatal maternal weight loss
- Postnatal visiting schedule based on individual needs
- Offer family planning and contraceptive advice

Do not attempt this procedure unless criteria for safe delivery have been met (see Table)

INDICATIONS

Fetal

● Presumed fetal compromise developing in second stage

● Suspected fetal compromise

If fetal compromise suspected, confirmation using fetal blood sampling (FBS) is preferable before a difficult instrumental delivery

Maternal

● Medical indications (e.g. cardiac disease, cerebrovascular disease and hypertension)

Delay in second stage of labour

● See **Delay in labour** guideline

● In the absence of other concerns, maternal exhaustion, etc.

Other

● After-coming head of the breech

CONTRAINDICATIONS

● Vacuum extractor contraindicated with a face presentation

● **Avoid:**

○ use of vacuum <34 weeks' gestation because of preterm susceptibility to cephalohaemtoma, intracranial haemorrhage and neonatal jaundice

○ metal cups <36 weeks' gestation

○ forceps/vacuum extraction deliveries before full dilatation of cervix

CRITERIA FOR SAFE OPERATIVE VAGINAL DELIVERY

	Essential
Full abdominal and vaginal examination	● Head <1/5 palpable per abdomen ● Vertex presentation ● Cervix fully dilated and membranes ruptured ● Exact position of head determined so that instrument can be placed properly ● Pelvis deemed adequate ● Optimise contractions
Mother	● Clear explanation given and informed consent obtained and documented (including episiotomy) ● Continuous electronic fetal monitoring ● Appropriate analgesia in place: ○ regional block ○ pudendal block ○ local infiltration ● Maternal bladder emptied – consider use of in/out catheter or, if indwelling catheter *in situ*, deflate balloon (recommended practice) ● Aseptic technique
Staff	● Operator has been assessed as competent in the use of forceps and vacuum extractor ● Adequate facilities and back-up personnel must be available ● Back-up plan in place in case of failure to deliver ● Anticipation of complications (e.g. shoulder dystocia, postpartum haemorrhage) ● Personnel trained in neonatal resuscitation e.g. midwife or ANNP/neonatologist (according to local policy) are present

Issue 3
Issued: April 2015
Expires: April 2017

TRIAL OF OPERATIVE VAGINAL DELIVERY IN THEATRE

- If there is doubt as to whether instrumental delivery will succeed, conduct delivery as a trial of vaginal delivery in theatre where, should a caesarean section be required, theatre team and anaesthetist are present
- appropriately trained person must undertake or supervise in theatre
- Consider instrumental delivery in theatre particularly in the following situations:
- multiparous women; especially with a previous vaginal delivery
- mid-cavity deliveries or where head palpable in the abdomen
- position is not occipito-anterior
- obese women where assessment of fetal size is difficult
- there has been delay in labour despite oxytocin
- estimated fetal weight >4000 g

Higher rates of failure are associated with

- Maternal obesity BMI >30
- Clinically big baby/estimated fetal weight >4000 g
- Malposition
- Mid-cavity delivery

What instrument?

- Doctor should choose instrument most appropriate to clinical circumstances and their level of expertise. Forceps and vacuum extraction are associated with different benefits and risks:
- Ventouse associated with more neonatal trauma and higher risk of failure
- forceps associated with more perineal trauma and 3rd and 4th degree tears
- Kielland's forceps should be used only by those trained and assessed as competent in their use

Dual instrumental delivery

- Dual instrumental delivery is associated with an increased risk of trauma and neonatal morbidity
- If satisfactory descent and/or rotation achieved before displacement of the vacuum, it is acceptable to complete a delivery with outlet forceps
- Attempt when it is very likely that a vaginal delivery will be successful (e.g. good descent of head in the perineum and detachment of Ventouse cup)

When to abandon operative vaginal delivery

- When there is no evidence of progressive descent with each pull, or where delivery is not imminent following 3 pulls of correctly applied instrument (cup or forceps) by an experienced doctor
- If delivery is thought to be imminent, with head in the perineum, it may, after careful re-evaluation, be appropriate to await one more contraction
- Poor progress or descent or concerns about fetal wellbeing should indicate the need to abandon the procedure (even if an episiotomy has been performed) and perform a caesarean section for the safety of mother and baby

Incident reporting

- Adverse outcomes, including unsuccessful forceps/vacuum delivery should trigger an incident report as part of effective risk management process. Follow local incident reporting procedure
- Paired cord blood samples processed and recorded following all attempts at operative delivery – see **Umbilical cord sampling** guideline

DOCUMENTATION

- **Clearly document in maternal healthcare record:**
- informed consent obtained
- analgesia used
- maternal bladder catheterised
- Use of instruments:
- number of pulls
- descent of head
- number of cup detachments
- total cup application time
- Episiotomy/tear findings and repair technique
- Cord gas blood results
- Swabs, needles, tampons (if used) to be counted before and on completion of procedure
- Record of incident report (if local practice)

AFTERCARE

- Perform local VTE risk assessment
- Give regular analgesia. If no contraindications, consider paracetamol and diclofenac/ibuprofen
- Bladder management – see **Bladder care** guideline

FOLLOW-UP

- An obstetrician (ideally who performed delivery) should discuss procedure, management of any complications and future deliveries with mother

Issue 3
Issued: April 2015
Expires: April 2017

INDICATIONS

- Induction of labour after artificial rupture of membranes (ARM)

- Acceleration/stimulation of labour after pre-labour rupture of membranes (PROM)

- prostaglandin induction may be appropriate before this – see **Pre-labour rupture of membranes (PROM)** guideline

- Augmentation when rate of progress in labour is considered unsatisfactory – see **Delay in labour** guideline

- For prevention of postpartum haemorrhage following delivery where there is an increased risk of bleeding – see **Postpartum haemorrhage** guideline

Assessment before oxytocin

- Before commencing oxytocin, midwife must confirm presentation is cephalic and membranes are ruptured

> *Before commencing oxytocin on a multiparous woman for delay in labour, an obstetrician of at least middle grade (ST3–7 or equivalent e.g. staff grade, clinical fellow) status must personally assess woman and perform abdominal palpation and vaginal examination*

- If previous caesarean section, the use of oxytocin should be or have been discussed with a consultant

Contraindications

- Non-rupture of membranes

- there are rare exceptions but these are consultant decision only

> *Do not commence oxytocin within 6 hr of administration of prostaglandin gel or tablet or within 30 minutes of removal of Propess pessary to prevent hyperstimulation – see Induction of labour guideline*

Monitoring

- Monitor fetus by continuous electronic fetal monitoring (EFM)

- if EFM suspicious, middle grade obstetrician (ST3–7 or equivalent e.g. staff grade, clinical fellow) to review woman

- if EFM pathological, stop oxytocin until assessment by middle grade obstetrician (ST3–7 or equivalent e.g. staff grade, clinical fellow)

- Perform routine maternal observations – pulse, blood pressure and temperature and record in partogram

- Perform vaginal examination no later than 6 hr after start of oxytocin and record planned timing of next vaginal examination

- Record individual management plan in intrapartum notes

OXYTOCIN REGIMEN

- Administer oxytocin through an infusion pump or syringe driver using a Y connector. This acts as a non-return valve to minimise risk of oxytocin being forced up into a second infusion and flushed through later as a bolus

- Use local regimen for oxytocin

- Increase infusion rate at no more than 30 minute intervals and by no more than the steps in the table (overleaf), until contractions are adequate

- There should be no more than four or five contractions every 10 min

- Once contractions established, especially in a parous woman, it may be possible and desirable to stop the infusion. Experience in the use of oxytocin is to be valued – seek the advice of midwife co-ordinator and middle grade obstetrician (ST3–7 or equivalent e.g. staff grade, clinical fellow) or consultant early

Suggested regimen – or follow local practice	
Time after starting (minutes)	**Equivalent milliunits/min**
0	1
30	2
60	4
90	8
120	12
150	16
180	20

Hyperstimulation

● Stop oxytocin and call middle grade obstetrician (ST3–7 or equivalent e.g. staff grade, clinical fellow)

● If stopping oxytocin does not correct hyperstimulation, consider tocolysis with 250 microgram terbutaline SC

Issue 3
Issued: April 2015
Expires: April 2017

INTRODUCTION

- Perineal trauma may occur spontaneously during vaginal birth or by a surgical incision (episiotomy). It is possible to have an episiotomy and a spontaneous tear (for example, an episiotomy may extend into a third-degree tear)

- Over 85% of women who have a vaginal birth will sustain some degree of perineal trauma and of these 60–70% experience suturing

DEFINITION

Anterior perineal trauma
Injury to labia, anterior vagina, urethra or clitoris

Posterior perineal trauma
Injury to posterior vaginal wall, perineal muscles or anal sphincters – may include disruption of the anal epithelium

Classification of perineal tears
Midwife/doctor must identify the extent of perineal trauma and document it according to the agreed classification

Definition of spontaneous tears

First degree	Second degree	Third degree
• Injury to skin only	• Injury to perineum involving perineal muscles but not involving anal sphincter	• Injury to perineum involving anal sphincter complex • 3a: <50% of external anal sphincter (EAS) thickness torn • 3b: >50% of EAS thickness torn • 3c: EAS and internal anal sphincter (IAS) torn See also **Third and fourth degree perineal tears** guideline

PRINCIPLES OF REPAIR

- All women receive a systematic assessment of the perineum, vagina and rectum and an accurate evaluation of any trauma sustained

- Give clear information regarding the extent of perineal trauma sustained, and how and when to seek advice if problems occur

Initial assessment

- Explain what is planned and why
- Offer entonox
- Ensure good lighting
- Position woman comfortably with genital structures clearly visible
- Perform initial examination gently and with sensitivity immediately after birth
- if genital trauma identified, carry out further systematic assessment including a rectal examination

Systematic assessment

- Further explain what is planned and why
- Timing of systematic assessment should not interfere with mother-infant bonding unless bleeding requires urgent attention
- Check equipment and count swabs, tampons and needles before commencing procedure and count again following completion of repair
- Lithotomy is the usual position to allow adequate visual assessment of the degree of trauma and for the repair. Maintain this position only as long as necessary for assessment and repair
- Confirm effective local or regional analgesia in place. Up to 20 mL lidocaine 1% can be used
- Assess trauma visually (with good lighting) including structures involved, apex of injury and degree of bleeding
- Perform rectal examination to identify damage to the external or internal anal sphincter

Documentation

- Clearly document in maternal healthcare record:
- examination findings, using agreed classification above, consider using a diagram
- if rectal examination performed as part of initial assessment
- if rectal examination was not carried out and reasons for not doing so

Perineal suturing

Consent

- Explain procedure, obtain and record consent
- Women who refuse to be examined and/or decline perineal repair must be given the opportunity to discuss their concerns with the person providing care. Discussion should include information about the potential risks which may occur if trauma to the sphincters remains undetected
- ensure discussion is clearly documented

Equipment

- Suture pack
- Sterile gown and gloves
- Protective glasses
- Cleansing solution or sterile water
- Suture material – Vicryl Rapide 2–0 (or equivalent) on a 35 mm taper cut needle
- 10–20 mL syringe and green needle
- Obstetric cream
- Local anaesthetic – lidocaine 1% up to 20 mL. If more required, consider spinal anaesthetic
- Adequate lighting
- Drapes

Procedure

- Complex trauma must be repaired by an experienced obstetrician in theatre under regional or general anaesthesia

- Suture as soon as possible following delivery to reduce blood loss and risk of infection, except in women who have laboured in the pool or had a water birth, in which case, suture after an hour
- Use an aseptic technique
- If woman reports inadequate pain relief, provide immediately
- Ensure good anatomical alignment of the wound and give consideration to the cosmetic result
- Use a continuous non-locked suturing technique for the vaginal wall and muscle
- If skin is opposed following muscle suturing it is not necessary to suture it
- Where skin does require suturing use a continuous subcuticular technique
- Suture first degree tears unless edges are well opposed
- On completion of repair, perform further rectal examination to exclude any suture material inserted through rectal mucosa
- Unless contraindicated, administer diclofenac (Voltarol) 100 mg rectally

> *Before and after suturing, perform and document a two-person swab, tampon (if used), needle and instrument check. Be particularly vigilant if there is heavy bleeding, a change of operator or transfer to theatre*

- If a vaginal pack is left *in situ*, document and communicate via handover
- Ensure safe disposal of all equipment in accordance with local Trust policy and COSHH regulations
- Document nature of trauma, method of repair and swab, tampon, needle and instrument count
- Unless contraindicated, prescribe and administer pain relief
- Advise woman about diet, hygiene and the importance of pelvic floor exercises

Problems with perineum after discharge from hospital

- If GP or community midwife concerned about a woman's perineum they should refer her urgently to the maternity unit or to the perineal trauma clinic

INTRODUCTION

Haemorrhage is a significant cause of direct maternal death. Obstetric haemorrhage can become life-threatening

RECOGNITION AND ASSESSMENT

- Normal blood volume from 13/40 is approximately 100 mL/kg
- Acceptable blood loss at vaginal delivery is 500 mL
- Acceptable blood loss at caesarean section is 1000 mL

Primary postpartum haemorrhage

- Excessive blood loss at or after delivery of fetus (see above for volumes) in first 24 hr. Affects approximately 5% of all deliveries in the UK

Secondary postpartum haemorrhage

- Excessive blood loss from genital tract >24 hr after birth and within 12 weeks of delivery

Blood loss

Definition

- Loss of ≥500 mL of blood from genital tract within 24 hr of birth of baby
- **Minor:** 500–1000 mL
- **Major:** 1000–1500
- **Massive:** >1500

> **Blood loss >20% must be treated**

PREVENTION

Table 1: Risk factors

Antepartum	Intrapartum
● Hypertensive diseases in pregnancy	● Prolonged third stage
● Multiple pregnancy	● Augmented labour
● Previous PPH	● Operative vaginal delivery
● Placenta praevia	● Episiotomy
● Antepartum haemorrhage	● Caesarean section
● Obesity	● Shoulder dystocia
● Age >40 yr	● Big baby
● Anaemia	
● Polyhydramnios	

Table 2: Cause of haemorrhage (the four T's)

4 T's	Specific cause	Relative frequency
A – Tone	● Atonic uterus	70%
B – Trauma	● Cervical, vaginal or perineal lacerations ● Pelvic haematoma ● Inverted uterus ● Uterine rupture	20%
C – Tissue	● Retained tissue ● Invasive placenta (accreta)	10%
D – Thrombin	● Coagulopathies	1%

Prevention is better than cure – follow the following principles

- Women at increased risk of bleeding, active management of third stage advised

- Give oxytocic [either syntometrine (ergometrine and oxytocin) or oxytocin 10 units IM (unlicensed) or 5 units by slow IV bolus in third stage

IMMEDIATE MANAGEMENT (ALL PPH)

- **Summon help** – senior obstetrician, anaesthetist, senior midwife and ancillary staff if necessary

- Keep woman warm

- **Consider:**

- **A – AIRWAY** – check airway not compromised

- **B – BREATHING** – oxygenate with 15 L/min oxygen via face mask

- **C – CIRCULATION** – obtain venous access – insert large bore 14 or 16 gauge cannula and take bloods for FBC, clotting screen, group and save and crossmatch if required (see **Major haemorrhage** below)

- **Palpate uterus** for atony and commence fundal massage. Consider bimanual compression

- **If woman did not receive syntometrine for management of third stage** and has not been hypertensive, and has had BP checked since admission, give ergometrine 500 microgram IM

- If required, give an antiemetic

- **Empty bladder** to assist with uterine contraction

- **Commence oxytocin** infusion using local regimen for postpartum

- **Monitor** physiological observations as per local practice

- **Document** fluid balance

MASSIVE OBSTETRIC HAEMORRHAGE

- Simultaneously perform resuscitation, monitoring, arresting bleeding and communication

In first instance – follow management as above

- **Estimate blood loss** by direct observation of overt blood loss **AND** clinical signs of intra-abdominal blood loss

- **Summon help:**

- middle grade obstetrician (ST3–7 or equivalent e.g. staff grade, clinical fellow)

- anaesthetist

- senior midwives (e.g. midwife co-ordinator and another experienced midwife)

- other personnel (e.g. porter/auxiliary/ HCA to run errands etc)

Bloods

- Canulate (insert two 14 or 16 gauge venous cannulae – one in each arm) and take blood for:

- FBC

- APTT

- PT (INR)

- crossmatch (at least 4 units of packed red cells)

- Consider taking blood for APTT, PT (INR) and U&Es

- Clotting is particularly important if the bleeding has been over a period of time

Fluids and fluid balance

- **Give fluids** – one litre compound sodium lactate (Hartmann's) solution stat

- Follow with blood, colloid or crystalloid as indicated by availability, blood loss and woman's haemodynamic state

- Do not give more than 3.5 L clear fluids [up to 2 L compound sodium lactate (Hartmann's) solution and 1.5 L colloid] while waiting for blood

- Insert urinary catheter with hourly urinometer attached and maintain urine output >0.5 mL/kg/hr

Blood transfusion

- Use local trigger phrase for massive obstetric haemorrhage:
- when requesting blood products from the biomedical scientist for haematology
- when contacting porters
- to communicate the urgency of the need for blood products

- Prepare blood/fluid warmer(s) to use as soon as possible especially for blood products
- Transfuse crossmatched packed cells as required
- In a dire emergency, consider requesting type specific blood
- Fresh frozen plasma (FFP) usually required if four units of packed red cells are given
- Use your Trust's Massive haemorrhage protocol

Table 3: Blood product replacement

Blood product	Indication
Packed red cells	Give fully crossmatched blood if possible. If insufficient time, give type specific and, only as an absolute necessity, give O negative blood
Fresh frozen plasma (FFP)	Avoid dilutional coagulopathy by early and adequate use of FFP (and other blood products as required)
Platelets	Give when count <50 x 10^9/L or significant ongoing bleeding with a count of <75 x 10^9/L or on consultant haematologist advice
Cryoprecipitate	Give if fibrinogen levels ≤100 mg/L and on consultant haematologist advice
Recombinant factor VIIa	Give only on consultant haematologist advice – 90 microgram/kg repeated 2-hrly if necessary
Tranexamic acid IV	20 mg/kg

Oxygen

- 15 L/min oxygen via face mask initially, with woman lying flat

Monitoring

- Attach non-invasive blood pressure (NIBP) cuff
- Monitor and record hourly on HDU chart:
- BP
- pulse
- SpO_2 (maintain at >95%)
- respiratory rate
- urine output and fluid balance
- core temperature

Inform

For massive obstetric haemorrhage, use local trigger phrase to communicate the seriousness of the situation clearly

- Consultant obstetrician (who will usually attend as soon as possible)
- Consultant anaesthetist
- Theatre team (even if not immediately going to theatre)
- Haematology biomedical scientist to allow them to prepare for major haemorrhage

- Haematologist if:
- blood products other than 4 units of packed cells and 4 units of FFP are required, or
- if there is ongoing haemorrhage after this has been given or
- if clotting studies are abnormal
- Consider involving surgical colleagues as required

Specific treatment

- For causes of haemorrhage (4 Ts) including surgery – see **Tone (uterine atony), Trauma, Tissue and Thrombin** below
- commonest cause is uterine atony
- If surgery to be carried out for major PPH, it is usual to obtain consent for hysterectomy
- Involve consultant with greater gynaecological surgical experience in complex cases. If available locally, consider contacting interventional radiologist

Repeat blood tests

- FBC
- APTT, PT (INR), fibrinogen
- Ca^{2+}
- Blood gases including lactate

Reassess

- State of haemorrhage and woman's physiological state after initial resuscitation

Central venous and arterial lines

- If continuing haemorrhage (or haemorrhage >40 mL/kg) or need to go to theatre for second time, insert CVC and arterial lines (and monitor CVP and BP directly)
- Use early if cardiovascular system compromised by disease

Hypocalcaemia

- Suspect if massive (>10 units blood) transfusion with ongoing hypotension, check Ca^{2+}. Give 10–20 mL calcium gluconate 10% by IV infusion over 10 min. Ensure ECG monitoring when administering calcium gluconate

Support for woman and family

- Ideally, midwife should remain with woman and family throughout the emergency situation

POST EVENT

- As soon as practically possible after a massive haemorrhage, consultant obstetrician should counsel woman and her family providing explanation and significance of cause of haemorrhage

Thromboprophylaxis

- These women are at increased risk of thromboembolism, whilst being nursed in HDU, consider anti-embolic stockings and other methods of mechanical thromboprophylaxis
- Unless advised to be inappropriate by consultant obstetrician/anaesthetist, give low molecular weight heparin regardless of mode of delivery once bleeding has settled

Non steroidal anti-inflammatory drugs

- Contraindicated for at least 12 hr after haemorrhage has settled and platelet count and renal function are normal

Documentation

- Carefully document:
- Times
- Drugs, fluids and blood products administered
- Personnel
- Use of trigger phrase
- Complete incident forms as required

A TONE (UTERINE ATONY)

Immediate management

- Fundal massage, empty bladder and consider bimanual uterine massage
- **Oxytocin** – Start oxytocin infusion. Use local regimen for postpartum via volumetric pump
- Remember to inspect vulva, vagina and cervix for trauma/lacerations
- Consider a first or repeat dose of oxytocin 5 or 10 units by slow IV bolus IM (unlicensed), ergometrine 250 microgram IM with an antiemetic [contraindicated in pregnancy induced hypertension (PIH) or other significant cardiovascular disease], misoprostol 1000 microgram PR or 250 microgram carboprost (methyl prostaglandin F2 Hemabate®) IM or intramyometrially (unlicensed) May be repeated up to every 15 min to a maximum of 2 mg. It would be unusual to reach the maximum dose

Continuing bleeding

- If above measures fail to prevent ongoing or recurrent bleeding, suspect Trauma, Tissue (e.g. retained products of conception) or Thrombin (e.g. a coagulopathy)
- Consider surgical examination under anaesthesia
- if woman haemodynamically stable, use pre-existent regional (epidural) anaesthesia
- if woman not stable or (dilutional) coagulopathy present, use general anaesthesia
- If bleeding still not controlled, consider uterine cavity balloon tamponade, haemostatic brace suture, hysterectomy, uterine artery ligation/embolisation by an interventional radiologist
- A consultant obstetrician must be involved
- A second consultant opinion before hysterectomy can be helpful but hysterectomy should be performed sooner rather than later

B TRAUMA

Inverted uterus

- Degree of haemodynamic shock is often disproportionate to the volume of the haemorrhage
- Replace uterus as soon as possible using manual, hydrostatic or surgical methods
- Anticipate massive haemorrhage
- Some women may experience a vasovagal episode (hypotension and bradycardia) during uterine replacement
- Run an oxytocin infusion using local regimen for postpartum for at least 4 hr after replacement

Uterine rupture

- See **Uterine rupture** guideline

Perineal trauma

- See **Third and fourth degree perineal tears** guideline and **Perineal trauma suturing (tears and episiotomy)** guideline

Other

- Broad ligament haematoma
- Extra genital bleeding e.g. sub capsular liver rupture

C TISSUE

Retained placenta

- See **Retained placenta** guideline

Placenta accreta/increta/percreta

- See **Morbidly adherent placenta** guideline
- If attempts are made to separate adherent placenta (surgically/forcibly), expect massive haemorrhage
- If expected or actual haemorrhage, follow management plan for major obstetric haemorrhage
- One option, after consultant review, is to leave the placenta *in situ* and monitor woman very closely for signs of infection and bleeding in postnatal period

D THROMBIN

Inherited coagulopathies

- Several inherited conditions will give rise to excessive peripartum haemorrhage if incorrectly managed and not detected antenatally. **Seek advice from consultant haematologist at earliest opportunity** (ideally antenatally) about the investigation and treatment of these varied and uncommon conditions

Acquired coagulopathies

- Will often represent a form of **Disseminated Intravascular Coagulation** (DIC) and will usually result in continuing or worsening haemorrhage without blood product replacement therapy

- Suspect DIC in abruption, severe PIH, prolonged +/- infected retained fetus/ products of conception, amniotic fluid embolism or prolonged/untreated hypovolaemic shock

- FBC, PT, INR, APTT, and APTTR in the first instance in all those conditions where there is a known associated complication of DIC

- If platelet count <50 x 10^9/L or INR >1.6, check fibrinogen and fibrinogen degradation products (FDP) levels

- Give FFP, platelets, +/- cryoprecipitate as directed by investigations

- Seek advice of a consultant haematologist about treatment and further investigations

Issue 3
Issued: April 2015
Expires: April 2017

INTRODUCTION

- Assessment and management of disease unrelated to the pregnancy are altered by the pregnancy
- The need to consider two patients (mother plus fetus) may change treatment decisions
- Anatomical and physiological changes in pregnancy result in altered:
- clinical features during CVS and respiratory system and abdominal examination
- biochemical and haematological values
- pharmacological management
- response to any systemic pathology
- protocols for the management of critical illness

AIM

- To ensure
- every pregnant woman admitted is managed promptly
- communication link is established between admitting team and obstetric team so that the most appropriate care can be delivered

ACTIONS

Accident and emergency

- Ask apparently pregnant woman presenting to Emergency department for any reason (irrelevant of gestation) if she has booked for maternity care
- if not booked for maternity care, inform delivery suite co-ordinator, who can advise on appropriate follow-up and booking arrangements
- In cases of trauma or bleeding at any gestation, give consideration to woman's blood group and need for Anti-D. If in doubt, discuss with on-call middle grade obstetrician (ST3–7 or equivalent e.g. staff grade, clinical fellow)

Nursing

- To prevent aortocaval compression, do not nurse women in the second and third trimester in supine position
- If the disease causes reduced mobility, consider VTE prophylaxis. Use local obstetric VTE assessment tool
- Use early warning scoring system (MEWS) to help in the timely recognition, treatment and referral of women who have or are developing critical conditions

Contact

- If any pregnant woman is admitted outside the maternity service you must contact:
- on-call middle grade obstetrician (ST3–7 or equivalent e.g. staff grade, clinical fellow) /consultant obstetrician
- if she is critically ill, or likely to need urgent surgery, refer early to the critical care team and/or anaesthetist
- if her gestation is ≥16 weeks, contact delivery suite co-ordinator, who will advise which healthcare professional(s) should review
- By giving consideration to the pregnancy and the fetus, the maternity service providers can help with:
- assessment of maternal and fetal wellbeing
- investigations
- treatment

> *Radiological investigations are not contraindicated during pregnancy where there is a significant clinical indication. Discuss with obstetric team*

Documentation

- Document all communication (including inter-departmental) in maternal healthcare record, highlighting pregnant or newly delivered woman's attendance or admission to non-midwifery ward or department

RECOGNITION AND ASSESSMENT

- Rupture of membranes before onset of labour ≥37 weeks' gestation
- majority of women will labour spontaneously within 24 hr of PROM
- PROM is associated with an increased risk of intrauterine infection

Risk factors for intrauterine infection

- Maternal group B *streptococcus* status
- Presence of meconium in amniotic fluid
- Increasing time from rupture
- Number of vaginal examinations
- Use of internal monitoring
- Length of labour and mode of delivery

Examination

- Full antenatal assessment, including fetal and maternal observations and abdominal palpation to confirm fetal lie and presentation
- Assess fetal wellbeing
- Speculum examination or pad test (if used locally) is only required if there is doubt about whether membranes have ruptured
- If contractions absent, do not perform digital vaginal examination, unless result necessary to guide or alter management
- Electronic fetal monitoring (EFM) 24 hr after PROM or earlier if other indications e.g. decreased fetal movement

Assessment and indications for immediate induction of labour (IOL)

- When forming management plan, determine if immediate induction of labour is necessary – see below
- consider duration of ruptured membranes

Indications for immediate induction of labour

- Induce labour immediately if:
- maternal pyrexia
- fetal distress
- significant meconium stained liquor
- blood stained liquor
- requiring Group B *streptococcus* prophylaxis
- HIV positive mother
- unstable presenting part
- maternal choice

MANAGEMENT

> *As time between rupture of membranes and onset of labour increases, so does the risk of maternal and fetal infection*

Expectant management

- Until IOL commenced or if woman chooses expectant management beyond 24 hr, care can be in-patient or out-patient
- If labour not started after 24 hr of ruptured membranes, arrange induction
- Record temperature 4-hrly during waking hours
- Woman to report immediately any change in temperature, colour or odour of amniotic fluid, any change in fetal movement pattern or if labour begins
- If any fever or change in colour or odour of amniotic fluid, commence induction
- Bathing or showering not contraindicated
- Sexual intercourse is contraindicated
- Provide woman with information leaflet before discharge home

Issue 3
Issued: April 2015
Expires: April 2017

Evidence of infection in mother

- Prescribe broad spectrum antibiotics – as per local practice

- Babies born with symptoms of possible sepsis or to a woman with evidence of chorioamnionitis, immediate referral to neonatologist (see **Group B streptococcus** guideline)

Induction and delivery

- Discuss with woman and explain procedure

- Use either oxytocin or prostaglandin

- On admission, perform digital vaginal examination using aseptic technique

- if cervix not ready for induction, use prostaglandin (see **Induction of labour** guideline) – follow local practice

- If local practice, consider antibiotic prophylaxis

- After 24 hr from membrane rupture, perform EFM

- Perform EFM in labour

POSTNATAL

- If delivery >24 hr following PROM, advise woman to remain in hospital with her baby for at least 12 hr following delivery

- Advise woman with PROM to inform midwife/GP immediately if concerned about baby's wellbeing in first 5 days following delivery, particularly in first 24 hr when risk of infection is greatest

Observations (baby)

- Perform Neonatal Early Warning Score (NEWS) observations

INTRODUCTION

- Although preterm is defined as delivery <37 completed weeks' gestation, most morbidity and mortality occur with delivery <34 completed weeks' gestation
- Diagnosis and prevention of preterm delivery is important as a means of reducing adverse outcomes for the baby
- for babies delivered >34 weeks' gestation, outcome is extremely good and labour is usually allowed to proceed
- for some women, tocolysis is inappropriate, e.g. labour too advanced, concerns about fetal infection or evidence of placental abruption
- Not all women presenting with symptoms of preterm labour will deliver preterm

Risk factors for preterm birth

- Previous preterm delivery
- Genital tract infection/inflammation
- Cervical weakness
- Uterine abnormalities
- Multiple pregnancy
- Polyhydramnios
- Bleeding/thrombosis
- Substance abuse
- Low body mass index (BMI)
- Short conception cycle <1 yr
- Age <17 yr or >35 yr

Diagnosis

- Diagnosis is difficult and is often wrong (50% of cases)
- For a reliable diagnosis of preterm labour, there should be painful uterine contractions >1 every 10 min, **plus** one or more of the following cervical signs:
- objective evidence of cervical change over 2 hr minimum
- ruptured membranes
- preterm laboratory prediction test (e.g. actim partus, fetal fibronectin)

ASSESSMENT

- On-call middle grade obstetrician assesses all women with suspected preterm labour or preterm ruptured membranes
- Maternal temperature, pulse, respiratory rate and blood pressure and MEWS
- Check gestation carefully
- Abdominal palpation to determine presentation. If in doubt, obstetric middle grade to confirm using labour ward portable ultrasound
- Palpate contractions to assess strength and frequency. Note any tenderness
- Perform electronic fetal monitoring (EFM) – continue this while contracting regularly
- Perform sterile speculum examination without lubricant except sterile water
- if appropriate (see below), perform preterm laboratory prediction test (e.g. actim partus, fetal fibronectin) **first**
- HVS, endocervical swab in Stuarts medium and endocervical swab for chlamydia
- MSU, FBC and CRP

Digital examination

- Digital examination, performed by obstetric middle grade or consultant, is only indicated when regular contractions have been palpated or after an abnormal speculum examination

> *Digital examination can introduce infection and release prostaglandins and should be avoided in preterm rupture of membranes without contractions*

Preterm laboratory prediction testing (e.g. actim partus, fetal fibronectin)

- Valid only between 23–35 weeks' gestation
- Test not indicated if:
- evidence of membrane rupture
- moderate or gross bleeding
- placenta praevia or abruption suspected
- To reduce risk of false positive result, do not use lubricant (other than sterile water) for speculum examination
- Take swab from posterior fornix before any other vaginal or cervical swab or digital examination
- If sexual intercourse occurred in previous 24 hr, test may be difficult to interpret

Issue 3
Issued: April 2015
Expires: April 2017

FFN value ng/mL	% who will deliver within 2 weeks	% who will deliver <34/40	Suggested management
0–9	<2	<2	Routine home follow up
10–49		5–15	Routine home follow up
50–199	5–15	10–15	Admit Betamethasone Consultant-led care
200–499	30	30	Admit Betamethasone with tocolysis $MgSO_4$ if <30/40 Consultant-led care Consider repeat FFN in ANC
>500	50	75	Admit Betamethasone with tocolysis $MgSO_4$ if <30/40 Consultant-led care

COMMUNICATION

- Discuss all aspects of care with woman and her partner
- Discuss and clearly document any change in plan
- Liaise with neonatal team
- Ensure parents spoken to by a senior neonatologist

MANAGEMENT OF <23 WEEKS' GESTATION

- Unless there is uncertainty about gestational age, care for woman as a late miscarriage

MANAGEMENT OF ≥23 WEEKS' GESTATION

- See **Flowchart** and formulate a clear management plan including:
  - steroids
  - tocolysis
  - antibiotics
  - mode of delivery
  - type of fetal monitoring
  - communication

Use of steroids, tocolysis and antibiotics

Membranes	Cervix	Preterm laboratory prediction test	Initiate steroids	Initiate tocolysis	Initiate antibiotics
Intact	≤4 cm	Positive	Yes	Yes	No
Ruptured	≤4 cm	NOT required	Yes	Yes	Yes
Intact or ruptured	>4 cm	NOT required	If delivery not imminent, yes	No	If ruptured membranes, yes

Steroids

- Consultant obstetrician decides on use of steroids if:
  - signs of infection
  - diabetic mother
  - steroids already given earlier in pregnancy
  - 23+0–23+6 week' gestation
- Otherwise, prescribe betamethasone when there is a significant risk of premature delivery between 24–35 weeks' gestation
  - if appropriate, administer two 12 mg doses IM 12 or 24 hr apart (depending on clinical situation) to promote fetal lung maturity

Tocolysis

- Use as indicated in Table **only** to allow time for steroids to act or for transfer to another unit
- Use only if cervix ≤4 cm dilated, **and** either membranes ruptured or vaginal preterm laboratory prediction test (e.g. actim partus, fetal fibronectin)
  - it is usually futile to start tocolysis beyond >4 cm dilatation with a fully effaced cervix
  - tocolytics are contraindicated in antepartum haemorrhage or suspicion of intrauterine sepsis **or** where baby would be safer delivered
- Site IV line with crystalloid solution running in all women receiving tocolytics in case of sudden change in blood pressure
- Record pulse and blood pressure before each dose of tocolytics (e.g. atosiban, nifedipine – see **Regimens** below)
- Atosiban and nifedipine are equally effective in delaying delivery. Atosiban has a more favourable side effect profile but is considerably more expensive

Cot availability

- Call neonatal unit to check availability of neonatal cot
- If no cot available, consultant obstetrician will decide whether to transfer mother to a unit with neonatal cot
  - check availability of cots in local network
  - contact labour ward of receiving unit to confirm they can accept the woman. See **Maternal transfer** guideline

PRETERM RUPTURE OF MEMBRANES IN THE ABSENCE OF CONTRACTIONS

- Manage as above
- **Do not** carry out digital examination
- Assess risk of cord prolapse – see **Umbilical cord prolapse** guideline
- Unless signs of infection or any other indication that fetus would be safer delivered, admit woman to antenatal ward
- Commence oral erythromycin 250 mg 6-hrly for 10 days to reduce risk of preterm labour and delivery. Consultant obstetrician decides whether to extend the use of erythromycin beyond 10 days
- If woman pyrexial, erythromycin will not provide cover for Gram negative and anaerobic infections. Commence antibiotics to cover Gram positive, Gram negative and anaerobic organisms, e.g. cefuroxime and metronidazole – follow local policy
- If 34–37 weeks' gestation, discuss induction of labour with consultant
  - immediate induction may be appropriate for GBS colonised women

23–26 WEEKS' GESTATION

- See also **Extreme prematurity** guideline
- Babies delivered <26 weeks' gestation have a high morbidity and mortality rate. Discuss how labour should be managed with consultant obstetrician and mother

- Manage as outlined with the following differences:
- it may not be appropriate to monitor fetal heart in first stage of labour, particularly if no action would be taken in the event of abnormalities. Consider fetal monitoring in second stage as this may influence management and may be of importance to neonatologist in considering resuscitation
- it may be appropriate to deliver baby vaginally, regardless of presentation. Consultant obstetrician must make decision to undertake a caesarean section at this gestation and should normally attend
- neonatal middle grade attends delivery

<30 WEEKS' GESTATION

Magnesium sulphate

- Magnesium sulphate protects premature babies' brains from cerebral palsy
- Consider for all babies likely to deliver in the next 24 hrs before 30 weeks' gestation regardless of mode of delivery. It can be given to women with multiple pregnancy and irrespective of whether steroids have been given
- Ideally, commence infusion 4 hr before delivery but if given <4 hr before delivery may still be beneficial
- Do not delay delivery in time-critical situations e.g. fetal distress
- administration may also be impractical when delivery is imminent
- The decision to administer magnesium sulphate must be made by a consultant obstetrician
- If woman did not deliver as expected, a repeat dose can be given later in the pregnancy
- Inform woman about possible side effects. The most common of which are:
- facial flushing
- nausea and vomiting
- sweating
- tachycardia and hypotension have also been observed
- The effect may be more pronounced when given with calcium channel blockers e.g. nifedipine

Loading dose

- Administer 4 g (8 mL) IV
- mix 4 g (8 mL) magnesium sulphate 50% with 12 mL sodium chloride 0.9% (total of 20 mL)
- set syringe driver at 60 mL/hr and administer over 20 min

Maintenance dose

- Administer 1 g/hr IV via syringe pump until delivery or for 24 hr, whichever is sooner
- mix 5 g (10 mL) magnesium sulphate 50% with 40 mL sodium chloride 0.9% (total of 50 mL)
- set syringe driver to 10 mL/hr and administer at 1 g/hr

Monitoring

- Oxygen saturation continuously with a pulse oximeter
- Hourly respiratory rate, blood pressure and level of consciousness
- Monitor deep tendon reflexes according to local protocol
- Check reflexes more often when there is oliguria, woman is also taking nifedipine and dose of magnesium sulphate has needed adjustment
- Stop infusion immediately and call middle grade obstetrician if:
- tendon reflexes absent
- respiration <12/min
- SpO_2 <95%
- abnormal conscious level
- urine output <1.5 mL/kg over 4 hr

Antidote

- 1 g (10 mL 10% solution) calcium gluconate IV over 3 min

LABOUR AND DELIVERY

- Decide mode of delivery on an individual basis. In general, if presentation not cephalic and once labour confirmed, delivery will be by caesarean section
- Electronic fetal monitoring
- **after 26 weeks' gestation** – throughout labour to assess fetal wellbeing
- **<26 weeks' gestation** – on the direction of obstetric consultant. See **Extreme prematurity** guideline
- Ensure delivery room/theatre warm. Shut windows, turn off fans and turn on resuscitaire heater well before delivery – premature babies are vulnerable to hypothermia
- Prematurity is an intrapartum risk factor for early onset Group B Streptococcus (GBS). Follow local policy for the use of antibiotic prophylaxis in labour
- Episiotomy is indicated to prevent delay in second stage of labour. There is no evidence that routine episiotomy prevents intracranial haemorrhage
- If <34 weeks' gestation and it is necessary to accelerate delivery, Ventouse is contraindicated
- At vaginal births, if possible, delay cord clamping for at least 30–45 seconds with baby held below mother to promote placento-fetal transfusion
- Neonatal middle grade and junior doctor attend delivery of <32 weeks' gestation
- Remember to put a hat on baby
- <29 weeks' gestation, place baby in a polythene bag on the resuscitaire to reduce risk of hypothermia
- Obtain paired cord blood samples for blood gas analysis and inform neonatal unit of results – see **Umbilical cord sampling** guideline

ATOSIBAN REGIMEN

Initial treatment

- Bolus dose 6.75 mg over 1 min
- Comes ready prepared as a 0.9 mL IV injection containing 6.75 mg, and can be diluted with sodium chloride 0.9% to make infusion over 1 min easier

Subsequent treatment up to 48 hr – via infusion pump

- Remove and discard 10 mL from a 100 mL bag of sodium chloride 0.9%. Add 2 x 5 mL vials of atosiban (37.5 mg total) to make a solution of 0.75 mg/mL
- Infuse 18 mg/hr for 3 hr (24 mL/hr for 3 hr)
- Then infuse 6 mg/hr for a maximum of 45 hr (8 mL/hr for maximum of 45 hr). Discontinue if contractions cease
- Total maximum duration of therapy 48 hr, total maximum dose given 330 mg

Routine obstetric observations

- Continuous EFM
- Strict fluid balance, though no specific restrictions
- Monitor blood loss after delivery

NIFEDIPINE REGIMEN

Contraindications

- Aortic stenosis
- Heart failure
- Porphyria
- Severe hypotension

Initial treatment

- 20 mg nifedipine **capsule (do not crush)** or slow-release tablet dispersed in water

Observations

- BP every 15 min for first 2 hr after first dose and once 15 min after subsequent doses
- Nifedipine should not cause a drop in blood pressure in normotensive women
- Continuous electronic fetal monitoring for first 2 hr

Subsequent treatment up to 72 hr

- 10–20 mg nifedipine retard **(slow release tablet)** 8-hrly adjusted according to uterine activity

Issue 3
Issued: April 2015
Expires: April 2017

Flowchart for management of preterm labour up to 34 weeks' gestation

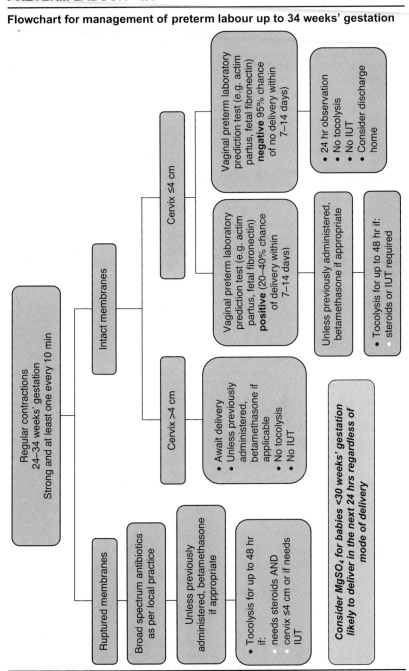

Regular contractions
24–34 weeks' gestation
Strong and at least one every 10 min

Intact membranes

Cervix >4 cm
- Await delivery
- Unless previously administered, betamethasone if applicable
- No tocolysis
- No IUT

Cervix ≤4 cm

Vaginal preterm laboratory prediction test (e.g. actim partus, fetal fibronectin) **positive** (20–40% chance of delivery within 7–14 days)
- Unless previously administered, betamethasone if appropriate
- Tocolysis for up to 48 hr if: steroids or IUT required

Vaginal preterm laboratory prediction test (e.g. actim partus, fetal fibronectin) **negative** 95% chance of no delivery within 7–14 days)
- 24 hr observation
- No tocolysis
- No IUT
- Consider discharge home

Ruptured membranes
- Broad spectrum antibiotics as per local practice
- Unless previously administered, betamethasone if appropriate
- Tocolysis for up to 48 hr if:
  - needs steroids AND
  - cervix ≤4 cm or if needs IUT

Consider MgSO₄ for babies <30 weeks' gestation likely to deliver in the next 24 hrs regardless of mode of delivery

STAFFING

- Recovery staff (ODP, midwife or nurse) must be appropriately trained to the standard required for general recovery facilities

- To ensure competency is maintained, staff should work in the general theatre recovery unit regularly and have access to CPD and mandatory training

- Observe all women on a one-to-one basis

Equipment

- Ensure appropriate equipment is available in recovery room and meets Association of anaesthetists of Great Britain and Ireland (AAGBI) requirements

POST-ANAESTHETIC CARE

- Begins as soon as surgical procedure completed

- Woman must be physiologically stable on departure from operating theatre

- Anaesthetist must determine need for monitoring during transfer

- Following extubation in theatre, transfer woman to recovery room

- Anaesthetist formally hands over care to recovery room nurse, operating department practitioner (ODP) or appropriately trained midwife but remains responsible for the woman and must be readily contactable

- One-to-one care

- Woman remains in recovery room for a minimum of 30 min or until discharge criteria met – see below

- Midwifery care is required

- to assess fundal height and lochia

- to commence skin-to-skin contact and offer help with first breast feed

- If woman conscious, birth partner can accompany her to recovery

MONITORING AND DISCHARGE CRITERIA (RECOVERY ROOM)

Mother

- Monitor and record on local documentation

- For all women, monitor the following parameters at least every 10 min, as a minimum:

- heart rate

- blood pressure

- SpO_2

- respiratory rate

- temperature once

- Other parameters that may need to be monitored and that must be assessed before discharge are listed in **Tables** overleaf

MONITOR	DISCHARGE CRITERIA
General	
Temperature	36–37.5°C
Airway	Able to breath deeply and cough on command
Blood glucose – if appropriate	
Urinary output – amount and colour	Adequate and clear

● IV infusion running:
  type of fluid
  rate of administration	

Respiratory status	
SpO_2	Between 94–98% with room air or supplemental oxygen
Respiratory rate	Between 10–20/min

Cardiovascular status	
Pulse rate	50–100 beats/min. No unexplained cardiac arrhythmias
Systolic blood pressure	Within 20% of pre-anaesthetic level

Neurological status	
Conscious state	Easily rousable and able to respond appropriately to questions

Motor status	● Able to:
	  sustain head lift for minimum of 5 sec
	  move limbs in a co-ordinated manner
	  signs of motor recovery

Post-surgical status	
Surgical drainage	● No active signs of blood loss from wound/drainage sites/vagina ● Acceptable fundal height

Pain control if opioids administered – 20 min observations	
● Pain assessment ● Analgesia administered and documented	Woman must be pain-free or acknowledge pain score ≤3 or mild

Post-operative nausea and vomiting (PONV)	
Document treatment for PONV and effectiveness, e.g. treatment sheet, healthcare record	Must be controlled before discharge to ward

Personal hygiene	
Check	Ensure woman clean, dry and comfortable

Baby

- See **Care of the newborn at delivery** guideline

- If woman conscious and baby well, hand baby to her immediately. Encourage skin-to-skin

DISCHARGE FROM RECOVERY

- If discharge criteria not achieved, keep woman in recovery room and inform anaesthetist who must review

Unsuitable for transfer to postnatal ward

- May require further intensive observations on delivery suite following assessment by anaesthetist and middle grade obstetrician (ST3–7 or equivalent e.g. staff grade, clinical fellow)

- Frequency of observations will depend on woman's condition

Documentation

- **Must be completed and accompany woman on discharge:**
- clinical notes
- nursing record, midwifery notes
- post anaesthetic care record
- operation notes
- anaesthetic record
- treatment sheet/drug chart
- fluid infusion chart

CARE DURING 24 HOURS FOLLOWING RECOVERY

- Use this guideline in conjunction with your local Maternity Early Warning Scoring system (MEWS)

On postnatal ward

- Close monitoring during first 24 hr. If available at your Trust, nurse in a four-bedded room

- Intensity and frequency of observations will depend upon:
- stage of recovery
- nature of surgery
- clinical condition of woman
- type of analgesia [e.g. PCA i.e. intrathecal opioids (diamorphine)]

Observations on ward

- On admission, perform initial assessment:
- BP
- pulse
- oxygen saturation levels
- respiratory rate
- temperature
- conscious level
- Assess the following as appropriate:
- surgical site and drains
- vaginal loss
- palpate uterine fundus
- catheter bag drainage – urine output
- IV infusions
- pain and sedation levels
- nausea and vomiting

Issue 3
Issued: April 2015
Expires: April 2017

GENERAL PRINCIPLES

Consent

- Transfusion without consent is a gross physical violation – follow your local Trust **Consent** policy

Mentally competent women

Aged ≥18 yrs

- Have a fundamental legal and ethical right to refuse treatment (including blood transfusions) even if it is likely that refusal will result in their death
- No other person is legally able to consent to treatment for that adult or to refuse treatment on their behalf
- Administration of blood or blood products to a competent adult without consent or against their wishes is unlawful and ethically unacceptable and may lead to criminal, civil or disciplinary proceedings
- Women may refuse blood transfusions for many reasons, including:
- religion
- safety concerns
- previous transfusion reactions
- previous negative experience

Aged <18 yrs

- In law women aged 16–18 yrs have the same capacity and right to consent to treatment as persons aged ≥18 yrs. Case law has extended the right to persons aged <16 yrs who are judged to have the capacity to fully understand what is proposed
- Where a woman aged <16 yrs is believed to have the necessary capacity, her acceptance of treatment cannot be nullified by parental objection
- Where a woman aged <16 yrs refuses blood products, seek urgent advice from Trust manager/director on-call. Consider second opinion from consultant obstetrician/anaesthetist/haematologist

Unconscious/incapable woman

- If an unconscious or apparently incapable woman is admitted, treat in the normal way, except where:
- there is compelling evidence that the person, if capable, would refuse to accept blood (e.g. carrying a card or document rejecting blood transfusion in all circumstances, especially if noted at booking). Her wishes must be respected provided the decision is clearly applicable to the present circumstances and there is no reason to believe she has changed her mind
- Views of close relatives or friends could be taken into account but would not be decisive (General Medical Council 1998)
- in cases of dispute, seek urgent advice from on-call consultant haematologist and Trust manager/director on-call

AT BOOKING

Discussion and documentation

- Ask all women if they have any objection to blood transfusion – document response
- Wherever possible, see woman on her own without outside influence
- discuss risks of refusing blood e.g. may be life-threatening if massive haemorrhage
- Document conversation and woman's decision in maternal healthcare record
- If available at your Trust, give her a 'Receiving a blood transfusion' leaflet

Refusal

- If woman does not wish to accept blood transfusions in any circumstances, ask her to complete an advance directive/decision to this effect. Place one copy in maternal healthcare record and the other in main case notes
- Complete a neonatal alert/maternal alert form and any other alert system used locally
- Refer her to consultant obstetrician and consultant anaesthetist

Investigations and preparation

- Check blood group, antibody status, haemoglobin and serum ferritin
- start ferrous sulphate and folate to be given throughout pregnancy to maximise iron store
- Ultrasound scan to identify placental site

ANTENATAL

- Prepare a detailed birth management plan with woman
- She must be informed of services available e.g. cell salvage, haemodilutation and interventional radiology
- Aggressively manage anaemia
- in anaemia, consider erythropoietin after discussion with haematologist
- If unusual bleeding occurs at any time during pregnancy, advise woman to attend hospital for review by a middle grade obstetrician (ST3–7 or equivalent e.g. staff grade, clinical fellow), If actively bleeding, on-call obstetric consultant will be informed. Threshold for intervention will be lower than in any other woman
- Bleeding must be quantified as accurately as possible
- In the event of a significant haemorrhage, involve duty consultant anaesthetist and on-call consultant haematologist in management
- If high blood loss during caesarean section anticipated (e.g. placenta praevia), discuss at multidisciplinary level and make appropriate arrangements e.g. cell salvage

Reversal of decision

- If woman changes her decision in any way, complete a 'Reversal of advance decision' form (if available locally) and file in front of the Advance decision
- The maternal alert form will be updated to reflect this reversal of decision. All forms will remain in woman's healthcare record and will not be removed even if a reversal of advanced decision is made

LABOUR

- When a woman refusing blood transfusion is admitted, follow individualised management plan and inform consultant obstetrician and consultant anaesthetist on-call
- Routine labour management, by experienced staff
- Consent obtained for active third stage of labour – see **Third stage of labour** guideline

At delivery

- When baby delivered, give mother 1 mL Syntometrine IM
- Do not leave mother alone for at least 1 hour following delivery
- Monitor lochia closely for at least 1 hour after delivery
- If increased risk of postpartum haemorrhage, give 40 units oxytocin in 500 mL sodium chloride 0.9% by IV infusion pump as per local infusion regimen. This will include women with:
- history of bleeding (post or antenatal haemorrhage)
- prolonged labour especially if augmented with oxytocin
- maternal age >40 yrs
- four or more children
- multiple pregnancy
- large baby (>3.5 kg)
- maternal obesity
- polyhydramnios
- fibroids
- If baby transferred to neonatal unit, ensure neonatologists are aware of mother's views

CAESAREAN SECTION

- If caesarean section necessary, it must be carried out by senior obstetrician and senior anaesthetist

Elective surgery

- Inform consultant obstetrician and anaesthetist responsible for woman's care as soon as possible so they can meet with woman and discuss options

- Consider techniques available to reduce intra-operative blood loss, including:
- normovolaemic haemodilution
- intra-operative cell salvage
- tranexamic acid (if available locally)

TECHNIQUES FOR BLOOD CONSERVATION IN OBSTETRIC CARE

Acute normovolaemic haemodilutation (ANH)

- Immediate pre-operative collection of 2–3 units of whole blood from mother in citrated bags with simultaneous volume replacement with crystalloid/colloid to maintain normovolaemia
- Reduces the number of red cells lost at surgery
- Can be a primary means of conserving and re-transfusing platelets/coagulation factors – each unit of ANH blood is equivalent to 1 unit RBC + 1 unit FFP + 1.5–2 units of platelets

> *Do not suggest autologous blood storage to pregnant women, as the amount of blood required to treat massive obstetric haemorrhage is far in excess of that which could be donated during pregnancy*

Intra-operative cell salvage (ICS)

- Collection of blood from the operative field
- Collected blood is citrated, filtered, washed with sodium chloride, concentrated and returned to woman
- This technique requires specialist equipment and a dedicated perfusionist – see **Stem cell banking** guideline

MANAGEMENT OF HAEMORRHAGE

Post-operative care

- Give minimum 40% oxygen for 24 hr and manage in high dependency care area

- Monitor closely (including post-operative blood loss) and inform consultant obstetrician/surgeon immediately of any post-operative complications
- If admission to critical care likely, discuss with on-call critical care consultant
- In extreme cases, in order to lessen oxygen requirement, sedation, analgesia, IPPV with muscle relaxation and controlled hypothermia may be necessary
- Keep woman informed about what is happening

> *If any bleeding, act quickly. Inform consultant obstetrician and anaesthetist on-call.*
> *See Antepartum haemorrhage and Postpartum haemorrhage guidelines*

If standard treatment not controlling bleeding

- Strongly recommend blood transfusion. Woman is entitled to change her mind about a previously agreed treatment plan
- Staff must be satisfied that the woman is not being subjected to pressure from others. It is reasonable to ask accompanying persons to leave the room in order that a senior doctor (with midwife or other colleague) can confirm she is making the decision of her own free will
- If she maintains her refusal to accept blood or blood products, respect her wishes

Hysterectomy

- Early recourse to surgery may be necessary

DEATH

- See **Maternal death** guideline

DISCHARGE AND FOLLOW-UP

- Majority of pregnancies end without serious haemorrhage
- When discharging mother, advise her to report promptly if she has any concerns about bleeding during the puerperium

INTRODUCTION

- If placenta has not delivered or has shown no signs of separation 20 min after administration of syntometrine or oxytocin, prepare to treat promptly for retained placenta after 30 min
- If woman has requested a physiological third stage of labour and placenta has not delivered or shown signs of separation 60 min after birth, advise woman to allow active management of the third stage
- While waiting for placenta to separate, follow **Management** below

> ***Unnecessary delay increases risk of postpartum haemorrhage***

MANAGEMENT

- Monitor for shock and excessive blood loss
- Notify delivery suite co-ordinator that placenta has not delivered
- Encourage skin-to-skin/baby to breast
- Assist mother onto bed pan and encourage to empty bladder
- if unsuccessful, catheterise bladder
- Ensure mother is warm
- Ensure large bore IV cannula *in situ* and take blood for FBC and group and save
- Unclamp cord at maternal end to allow blood to drain out of the placenta once baby is detached
- Middle grade obstetrician (ST3–7 or equivalent e.g. staff grade, clinical fellow) will perform vaginal examination and check placenta not detached in vagina

> ***Do not attempt to remove an adherent placenta in delivery room or without anaesthetic***

- Manual removal of placenta takes priority over elective cases, even if woman not actively bleeding
- obstetric junior doctor can undertake this procedure under the direct supervision of a middle grade obstetrician (ST3–7 or equivalent e.g. staff grade, clinical fellow)

- if blood loss increases or maternal condition deteriorates, accelerate transfer to theatre
- Use gauntlets to protect the operator
- Midwife can accompany woman into theatre to support her throughout
- Administer broad spectrum IV antibiotics
- Following placenta removal, middle grade obstetrician (ST3–7 or equivalent e.g. staff grade, clinical fellow) must ensure uterus is empty
- Run oxytocin infusion for 4 hr after removal of placenta
- These women should stay on delivery suite for at least 2 hr
- Oral broad spectrum antibiotics for 5 days or as local practice
- In the case of postpartum haemorrhage – see **Postpartum haemorrhage** guideline

Communication

- Ensure woman and her partner, are fully informed at all times
- Obstetric middle grade obstetrician (ST3–7 or equivalent e.g. staff grade, clinical fellow) will see woman the following day to answer questions, especially in view of the uniquely penetrative nature of the procedure
- Inform woman of increased risk of placental retention in future pregnancy

Documentation

- Ensure clear and accurate documentation, including:
- procedure used
- total estimated blood loss since delivery

RETAINED PRODUCTS

- Where there is any concern about the completeness of delivered placenta, midwife must notify senior obstetrician regardless of mode of delivery
- Insert cannula, take blood for FBC and group and save
- Where there is a confirmed incomplete placenta, take woman to theatre for evacuation of retained products as above for a retained placenta

PRINCIPLES

● To encourage women to participate in planning postnatal care and to provide information to enable them to make informed choices

● To provide woman with relevant and timely information to enable her to recognise and respond to problems

● Lead professional will be responsible for postnatal period until woman and baby are discharged from midwifery care

Document all discussions in maternal healthcare record

POSTNATAL PERIOD

During in-patient episodes on delivery suite or postnatal ward, allocate woman and baby a named midwife for each shift, who will:

Maternal health	Infant health
● Ascertain physical and emotional health and wellbeing	● Enquire about baby's health
● Offer woman opportunity to talk about her birth experience and to ask questions about care received	● Provide information about:
◦ inform her about the debriefing service and how/who to contact if required	◦ promoting baby's health and general condition
● Discuss vaginal loss and perineal healing	◦ recognising signs and symptoms of common health problems in newborns and how to contact healthcare professionals as soon as a problem is suspected or in an emergency
● Look for signs and symptoms of mental health problems	● Advise woman to contact healthcare professionals if baby:
● Discuss coping strategies and support	◦ becomes jaundiced (or is jaundiced and it worsens)
● Encourage partner involvement	◦ passes pale stools
● Provide health promotion information and how to recognise life-threatening and common health problems – see **Life-threatening conditions in women** and **Common health problems in women** sections	● Provide advice and support on infant feeding
	◦ discuss breastfeeding and document any support required
● Confirm contact numbers (if woman is at home) and needs to report any concerns	● Give information regarding local support networks
● Women with physical, emotional, social or educational needs – see **Women with multiagency or multidisciplinary needs** section	● Check healthcare record for previous alerts
● Be alert to signs of domestic abuse. If concerned, follow local child protection and domestic abuse guidance	

● Midwives have direct access for referral to a consultant obstetrician at all times during the postnatal period if required

Women with multiagency or multidisciplinary needs

- Named midwife will:
  - co-ordinate woman's multiagency and multidisciplinary needs
  - liaise with named community midwife, lead midwife for vulnerable women and appropriate agencies and healthcare professionals
  - with woman's knowledge and, where possible and safe to do so, ensure appropriate agencies and healthcare professionals are involved according to local practice
  - document outcomes of multiagency or multidisciplinary meetings in woman's postnatal care plan

See also the following guidelines:

- Local **Safeguarding** guideline or local **Child protection** guideline
- Local **Mental health problems in pregnancy** guidance (if available)
- **Substance misuse** guideline
- Local **Management of domestic violence in pregnancy** guideline (if available)
- **Infant feeding** guideline

Initial postnatal period

- See **Care of the newborn at delivery** guideline
- Check woman's wellbeing, ensuring a minimum of one set of general observations have been taken and recorded and are within normal limits
- It is the responsibility of allocated midwife on postnatal ward to ensure it is safe to accept woman and/baby onto ward
- Ensure all allergies and sensitivities are documented
- Check baby is wearing 2 name bands containing woman's hospital number. Check this against mother's name band
- Assess general condition of baby
- Check that a birth weight has been performed and recorded in all relevant documentation

- Establish vitamin K has been administered and recorded
- Determine chosen method of feeding and obtain details of initial feed on delivery suite
- Commence red child health record book

Allocated midwife on postnatal ward will:

- See woman at each handover, review care plan and document in maternal healthcare record
- See **POSTNATAL PERIOD – At every postnatal contact** section at beginning of guideline
- See specific guidelines for appropriate care:
- **Infant feeding** guideline
- **Breastfeeding** guideline in the Staffordshire, Shropshire & Black Country Newborn and Maternity Network Neonatal guidelines (if used locally)
- **Hypoglycaemia** guideline in the Staffordshire, Shropshire & Black Country Newborn and Maternity Network Neonatal guidelines (if used locally)
- **Care of the newborn at delivery** guideline
- **Caesarean section** guideline
- **Bladder care** guideline
- **Group B streptococcal (GBS) disease** guideline
- **Pre-labour rupture of membranes** guideline
- **Substance misuse** guideline
- local **Transitional care** guideline (if available)
- **Hypothermia** guideline in the Staffordshire, Shropshire & Black Country Newborn and Maternity Network Neonatal guidelines (if used locally)
- **Jaundice** guideline in the Staffordshire, Shropshire & Black Country Newborn and Maternity Network Neonatal guidelines (if used locally)d locally)
- **Meconium stained liquor** guideline
- local **Administration of IV antibiotics** guideline, **Admission to SCBU** guideline and **Bed sharing** policy (if available)

Discharge home from delivery suite/birth unit

- Dependent upon individual circumstances and preferences, woman may choose to go home from delivery suite/birth unit or to be admitted to postnatal ward
- For home birth, see **Home birth** guideline

> *If woman or baby not considered appropriate for early discharge and woman insists on going home, complete a 'Discharge against medical advice' form*

Discharge directly following delivery	Discharge from delivery suite/birth unit/postnatal ward
• Provided no risk factor identified and no neonatal indication for admission, the following women may transfer home:	See also **POSTNATAL PERIOD – At every postnatal contact** section at beginning of guideline
normal, complication-free vaginal delivery	**Midwife will ensure:**
return of full mobility and 200 mL urine voided following epidural in labour	• Physical condition of mother and baby is satisfactory, and confirm identification of baby
insignificant meconium stained liquor in labour	• Referrals for mother and baby organised
any significant problem in previous pregnancy **not** affecting this birth e.g. previous retained placenta, third degree tear, instrumental delivery	• Woman's Hb, Rubella and Rhesus status have been checked and treated appropriately
walked to bathroom and passed urine – see **Bladder care** guideline	• Contraception has been discussed
• Discuss with team leader/middle grade obstetrician (ST3–7 or equivalent e.g. staff grade, clinical fellow)	• Smoking, including passive smoking and access to cessation of smoking programme for woman and other family members discussed
any mother who does not fit the above criteria but requests early transfer home. Discuss neonatal concerns with ANNP/neonatal staff	• Understanding of effective breastfeeding and, if planning to formula feed, correct preparation, sterilisation of equipment and storage of feeds discussed
	• Cot safety leaflet provided and discussed (if available locally)
	• Baby car seats discussed
	• Provide 24 hr contact number
	• Concerns relayed directly by postnatal midwife to community midwife
	• Inform woman that community midwife will visit the day after discharge and a subsequent visit will be arranged at that time
	ensure address documented is where the woman will be staying for first community visit, and confirm contact details are correct
	• Examination of newborn discussed (if not performed in hospital)
	• Parents advised how to register birth
	• File copy of discharge documentation
	• Woman has all relevant documentation, leaflets and prescribed medication

Postnatal visiting

Community midwife will:

- Visit woman at home on day following discharge and offer a minimum of 2 further postnatal contacts (day of delivery is day 0)

- **second contact:** day 5, to weigh baby and perform bloodspot test

- **third contact:** on or after day 10, to weigh baby and transfer care to GP and health visitor if appropriate

- date and venue to be agreed with woman. Can be at home or a drop-in clinic

- Discuss individual social, clinical and emotional needs, taking into account the views and beliefs of woman, her partner and family

- See also **POSTNATAL PERIOD – At every postnatal contact** section at beginning of guideline

> *Community team leader is responsible for ensuring all caseloads are picked up during periods of annual leave and/or sickness*

Newborn screening

- **It is the midwife's responsibility to:**

- discuss newborn screening with parents at least one day before being performed

- provide national screening committee leaflet 'Screening tests for your baby'

- obtain consent and take sample on day 5 (count date of birth as day 0). See **Bloodspot screening guideline** in the Staffordshire, Shropshire & Black Country Newborn and Maternity Network Neonatal guidelines (if used locally)

- ensure sufficient neonatal barcode labels available (if used locally) for when test is taken

- complete request card **after** performing test

- apply separate neonatal barcode label to each sheet of the card after checking details with parent(s)

- place specimen in correctly addressed envelope (use appropriate addressograph label)

- send to regional screening unit on day sample taken

- document according to local practice

- inform parents that health visitor will relay 'normal' results

- if any results abnormal or borderline, parents will be contacted directly

Preterm baby (<36 weeks' gestation)

- If baby almost 36 weeks' gestation, sample may be postponed for a few days to prevent unnecessary repeat

- Inform parents baby will need a repeat sample at 36 weeks corrected age for congenital hypothyroidism and arrange to visit and repeat test at the appropriate time

First 24 hours following initial delivery assessment

Woman's wellbeing	Baby's wellbeing and feeding
See also POSTNATAL PERIOD – At every postnatal contact section at beginning of guideline	

Midwife will:

- Discuss the following signs and symptoms of life-threatening conditions and how to contact their healthcare professional or call for emergency help:
  - sudden profuse blood loss
  - offensive/excessive vaginal loss
  - tender abdomen
  - fever
  - severe or persistent headache
  - raised BP with other signs of pre-eclampsia
  - chest pain and/or shortness of breath
  - unilateral calf pain/redness or swelling
- In first 6 hr following delivery, assess and document BP (see **Hypertension** guideline) and first urine void (see **Bladder care** guideline)
- Record maternal observations
- If offensive/excessive loss, abdominal tenderness or fever, assess vaginal loss, uterine involution and position
- Offer assessment of the perineum to any woman who suffered perineal trauma – see **Episiotomy** guideline, **Perineal trauma** guideline and **Third and fourth degree tears** guideline
- Ask about headache symptoms. If epidural or spinal used, advise woman to report headache, particularly if occurring while sitting or standing
- Assess thrombosis risk – see **VTE** guidelines and refer to obstetrician if appropriate
- Give woman opportunity to discuss the birth
- Encourage gentle mobilisation
- Give information on mental wellbeing
- Update postnatal care plan
- Ensure all contact numbers are clearly documented in maternal healthcare record and that woman and, if appropriate, partner/family also aware
- **Ensure all discussions clearly documented** in maternal healthcare record

Midwife will:

- Confirm and document urine passed
- Confirm meconium passed, if not, assess baby and seek medical opinion
- Ensure woman has received information regarding:
  - bathing – advise that cleansing agents, lotions and medicated wipes are not recommended in first 6 weeks
  - keeping the umbilical cord clean and dry (do not use antiseptic)
  - cot safety
  - parents aware of bed-sharing guidance from the Department of Health. The safest place for baby to sleep is in a cot in parents' room for first six months

Feeding

- Observe a full feed and offer ongoing feeding support
- Outline the benefits of colostrum and breastfeeding (this information should be culturally appropriate) – see **Breastfeeding** guideline in the Stafford, Shropshire & Black Country Newborn and Maternity Network Neonatal guidelines (if used locally)
- If artificial feeding, see **Infant feeding** guideline and Staffordshire, Shropshire & Black Country Newborn and Maternity Network Neonatal **Nutrition** guideline (if used locally)

Ensure all discussions/numbers given are clearly documented

Care in first week

Mother's wellbeing	Baby's wellbeing and feeding
See also POSTNATAL PERIOD – At every postnatal contact section at beginning of guideline	

Midwife will:

- Ensure Rh–D negative woman is offered Anti D immunoglobulin within 72 hr of delivering an Rh-D positive infant

- Within 3 days – discuss normal patterns of emotional changes in the postnatal period and that these usually resolve within 10–14 days

- Discuss the importance of appropriate exercise, rest and diet, including high fibre foods and adequate fluid intake

- If woman reports persistent fatigue, and suffered a postpartum haemorrhage, check Hb

- Offer information and reassurance on involuntary leakage of small amounts of urine commonly experienced after birth – see **Bladder care** guideline

- Advise woman to report concerns about haemorrhoids, rectal pain or bleeding, and if she has not opened her bowels within 3 days of delivery or regained her normal pattern

- Give perineal hygiene information

- Offer women with low-level or no immunity to Rubella on antenatal screening an MMR vaccination before discharge from maternity unit if possible. Can be given with Anti- D injection, provided separate syringe is used and administered into different limb

- if not given simultaneously, give MMR 3 months after Anti–D

- Advise woman to avoid pregnancy for 1 month after receiving MMR, but breastfeeding may continue

- Discuss future methods of contraception

- Look for changes in mood and emotional state, signs and symptoms of health problems, Seek information from family/partner if appropriate

- Observe for risks, signs and symptoms of domestic and child abuse and refer appropriately

- Update postnatal care plan using variances when required

Midwife will:

- Discuss all aspects of baby's physical health and wellbeing with parents, including continuous assessment of feeding

- Inform parents a full examination of baby will be performed within 72 hr of life and encourage them to be present. Provide full explanation including results of any tests

- Review family health history and address parental concerns

- Discuss neonatal screening

- Assess baby's general condition. Healthy babies should have normal colour for their ethnicity, maintain a stable body temperature and pass urine and stools at regular intervals

- Assess feeding behaviour – see **Infant feeding** guideline and **Breastfeeding, Nutrition** and **Hypoglycaemia** guidelines in the Staffordshire, Shropshire & Black Country Newborn and Maternity Network Neonatal guidelines (if used locally)

- Look for signs and symptoms of baby becoming unwell e.g. excessive irritability, tense, high temperature, sleepy or floppy

- Assess parent(s) for emotional attachment and offer information and support in adjusting to their new parenting role

- If any jaundice, record intensity, together with baby's hydration and alertness. If significantly jaundiced or unwell, inform medical staff and arrange evaluation of serum bilirubin level – see **Jaundice** guideline in the Staffordshire, Shropshire & Black Country Newborn and Maternity Network Neonatal guidelines (if used locally)

- provide parents information on, reason for and how to monitor jaundice (normally occurring around 3–4 days after birth)

- Weigh baby once within first week of life. If problem identified, more frequent weighing may be necessary

- If weight loss not within normal limits, inform parents and take appropriate action

- If parents concerned about baby's skin, advise to contact a healthcare professional

- Ensure bloodspot screening performed – see **Newborn screening** section and **Bloodspot screening** guideline in the Staffordshire, Shropshire & Black Country Newborn and Maternity Network Neonatal guidelines (if used locally)

- Explain bowel movement pattern in a normal neonate and inform parents to seek advice from healthcare professional if concerned about baby's bowel movements or urine output

- Update postnatal care plan, including variances where required and all discussions with parents

Issue 3
Issued: April 2015
Expires: April 2017

Life-threatening conditions in women	
Possible sign/symptom	**Evaluate for**
● Tachypnoea ● Sudden or profuse blood loss ● Blood loss and signs and symptoms of shock, including: tachycardia and hypotension hypoperfusion hypovolaemia change in consciousness	Postpartum haemorrhage (PPH) – see **Postpartum haemorrhage** guideline
● Offensive/excessive vaginal loss ● Tender abdomen or fever	PPH/sepsis/other pathology – see **Postpartum haemorrhage** guideline and **Sepsis** guideline
● Fever ● Shivering ● Abdominal pain ● Tachypnoea ● Offensive vaginal loss	Infection/genital tract sepsis
● Severe or persistent headache ● Diastolic BP >90 mmHg and other signs of pre-eclampsia	Pre-eclampsia/eclampsia – see **Eclampsia** guideline and **Severe pre-eclampsia** guideline
● Shortness of breath or chest pain	Pulmonary embolism
● Unilateral calf pain	Deep vein thrombosis

Common health problems in women	
Condition	**Action**
Baby blues	● If symptoms persist after 10–14 days, refer to GP for postnatal depression assessment

● Perineal pain
● Discomfort
● Stinging
● Offensive odour or dyspareunia
	● Perineal assessment and evaluate for signs of:
	  infection
	  inadequate repair
	  wound breakdown or non-healing
	● Refer as appropriate to GP/middle grade obstetrician (ST3–7 or equivalent e.g. staff grade, clinical fellow)
	● Advise topical use of cold therapy and paracetamol (if not contraindicated)
	  if neither effective, consider oral or rectal non-steroidal anti-inflammatory drug

Dyspareunia	● In cases of perineal trauma, offer perineal assessment (see above) if problems persist, refer to GP/ middle grade obstetrician (ST3–7 or equivalent e.g. staff grade, clinical fellow) for further evaluation
Headache	● Advise women who have had an epidural/spinal anaesthesia to report positional headache ● For tension/migraine headaches, offer advice on relaxation and avoiding precipitating factors
Persistent fatigue	● Ask about general wellbeing and provide advice on diet and exercise ● If condition affects woman's care of herself or baby, evaluate underlying causes ● Measure Hb and, if low, treat according to local practice
Backache	● Manage as general population
Constipation	● Assess diet and fluid intake if changes in diet ineffective, advise use of gentle laxative
Haemorrhoids	● If severe, swollen or prolapsed, evaluate and refer to GP for further evaluation/treatment otherwise, treat with haemorrhoid cream and provide advice on dietary measures to avoid constipation
Faecal incontinence	● Assess severity, duration and frequency. If symptoms do not resolve, refer to middle grade obstetrician (ST3–7 or equivalent e.g. staff grade, clinical fellow)/ incontinence nurse
Urinary incontinence	● Teach pelvic floor exercises ● If symptoms persist refer to incontinence nurse

Issue 3
Issued: April 2015
Expires: April 2017

Health problems in babies	
Problem	**Action**
Jaundice in first 24 hr	Refer urgently to paediatrician
Jaundice in babies aged >24 hr	Monitor and record jaundice and overall wellbeing, hydration and alertness
Jaundice in babies from 7 days of age or lasting >14 days	Refer to paediatrician
Significant jaundice or unwell babies	Evaluate serum bilirubin and refer to paediatrician
Jaundice in breastfed babies	Advise frequent feeding, waking baby to feed if necessary, routine supplementation is not recommended
Thrush	Offer information and guidance on hygiene. If appropriate, refer to GP for antifungal treatment
Nappy rash	Consider hygiene and skin care, sensitivity, infection, e.g. thrush
Persistent nappy rash	Refer to GP for consideration of antifungal medication
No meconium in first 24 hr	Refer to paediatrician urgently
Diarrhoea	Refer to paediatrician urgently
Excessive inconsolable crying	● Needs urgent action ● Reassure parents ● Assess general health: ◌ antenatal and perinatal history ◌ onset and length of crying ◌ nature of stools ◌ feeding ◌ woman's diet if breastfeeding ◌ family allergy ◌ parents' response ◌ factors that make crying better/worse
Colic	● Advise parents that holding baby during a crying episode and peer support may be helpful ● Do not use dicycloverine
Colic in formula-fed babies	Consider hypo-allergenic formula
Unwell baby	Refer urgently to paediatrician

Wellbeing and care in first 2–8 weeks

Mother's wellbeing	Baby's wellbeing and feeding
See also POSTNATAL PERIOD – At every postnatal contact section at beginning of guideline	

Midwife will:

- Ask woman about her physical, emotional and social wellbeing, and the wellbeing of her baby. Recognise symptoms that may need discussion/action
- Discuss resumption of sexual intercourse and possible dyspareunia
- Use routine screening questions for postnatal depression (within 10–14 days)
- Enquire about and give information on:
  - headache
  - perineal pain, discomfort, stinging, offensive odour or dyspareunia
  - persistent fatigue
  - backache
  - constipation
  - haemorrhoids
  - urinary or faecal incontinence
  - urine retention (within 6 hr of birth)
- Promote emotional attachment and improved parenting skills
- Provide information on local/national or voluntary groups that provide support and guidance in the postnatal period
- Discuss sudden infant death syndrome with parents, in line with DoH guidance
- Update postnatal care plan using variances when required. Document all discussions

Midwife will:

- Assess baby's feeding
- Provide advice and support woman's choice of feeding and document in postnatal plan
- Reinforce relevant safety issues for all family members in the home environment and promote safety education (e.g. safe sleeping). If parents choose to bed-share with baby, explain the increased risk of sudden infant death syndrome if either parent: smokes, has recently drunk alcohol, taken medication or drugs that make them sleep more heavily, or is very tired
- Discourage use of a dummy
- Discuss smoking, including passive smoking and access to cessation of smoking programme for woman and other family members if required
- Be alert to signs and symptoms of child abuse. If there are concerns, follow local child protection procedures
- Document all discussions in maternal healthcare record and baby healthcare record (red book)

Discharge from community midwifery care

- See also **POSTNATAL PERIOD, At every postnatal contact** section at beginning of guideline

Community midwife will:

- Assess physical/emotional and social wellbeing of mother and baby before discharge
- Discuss health issues e.g. breast awareness, cervical cytology, contraception and pre-conception advice
- Discuss arrangements for woman to attend for postnatal examination with GP approximately 6 weeks after birth
- Ensure necessary referrals for mother and baby have been completed

- Reinforce how to register baby's birth
- Discuss role of health visitor with parent(s)
- Complete necessary documentation in child healthcare record, to ensure comprehensive handover of care to health visitor
- Reinforce advice regarding local postnatal support/drop-ins/contact numbers and how to access them
- Ensure postnatal record completed and returned to hospital to enable maternal healthcare record to be filed and returned to medical records
- In all out of area deliveries, ensure midwifery postnatal records are returned to appropriate hospital as per local practice

BACKGROUND

- Sepsis is any suspected or known infection associated with a systemic inflammatory response

- Sepsis is a leading cause of maternal mortality in the UK and the most common cause of maternal mortality in the critical care unit (CCU)

- If septicaemic shock develops, mortality rates approach 60% in CCU

- Early detection, accurate diagnosis and aggressive appropriate treatment can significantly improve outcome

- One-third of women who die do so because of refractory hypotension whilst the rest die later from multi-organ failure

Risk factors for maternal sepsis

- Obesity

- Impaired glucose tolerance/diabetes

- Impaired immunity

- Anaemia

- Vaginal discharge

- History of pelvic infection

- Amniocentesis and other invasive intrauterine procedures

- Cervical cerclage

- Prolonged rupture of membranes (PROM)

- Vaginal trauma

- Caesarean section

- Wound haematoma

- Self or family history of, or contact with upper respiratory tract infection

- Group A *streptococcus* disease in close family/contacts

- Sickle cell disease/trait

- Black/ethnic minority

- Retained products of conception after miscarriage, termination of pregnancy or delivery

RECOGNITION AND ASSESSMENT

Symptoms, signs and laboratory results

> *Consider sepsis in any woman with symptoms and signs suggestive of abruption*

- Use a MEWS chart for all maternity in-patients to identify seriously ill pregnant women and refer them to critical care and obstetric anaesthetic colleagues according to local guidance

- Rigors, sweating, fever

- Headache, muscle pain, altered mental state, lethargy, poor appetite

- Features of primary infection. Consider especially genital tract sepsis (chorioamnionitis, postpartum endometritis); also wound infection, pyelonephritis, pneumonia, acute appendicitis, acute cholecystitis, pancreatitis, necrotising fasciitis, mastitis

- **An abnormal or absent fetal heart beat** with or without placental abruption may be the result of sepsis

- Sepsis is the presence of one of the above symptoms plus two of the following:

- heart rate >100 beats/min

- respiratory rate >20 breaths/min

- temperature >38°C or <36°C

- WBC >12 or <4 x 10^9/L – WBC normally raised in labour

- normal WCC with >10% immature forms or increased CRP

- hyperglycaemia in the absence of diabetes (plasma glucose >7.7 mmol/L)

- acutely altered mental state

Genital tract sepsis

- Vomiting and diarrhoea, and/or abdominal pain

- often attributed to gastroenteritis

- Vaginal discharge, wound infection

- Rash (generalised streptococcal maculopapular rash)

- discolouration or mottling of the skin may indicate cellulitis

Life-threatening features

- **Severe sepsis:** sepsis with impaired organ function [e.g. diminishing renal function, impaired cardiac function, hypoxia, acidosis, acute respiratory distress syndrome (ARDS), clotting disturbance, plasma lactate >4.0 mmol/L]

- **Septic shock:** severe sepsis with systolic BP <90 mmHg or MAP (mean arterial pressure) <65 mmHg

Investigations

Sepsis

- Swabs:

- vaginal

- endo-cervical (if swabs for chlamydia PCR, use chlamydia detection kit; if for N gonorrhoea culture, place swab in charcoal medium)

- wound

- throat

- FBC and differential WBC

- INR, APTT

- Group and save

- Biochemical screen (U&E, LFT and C-reactive protein)

- Glucose

- Culture

- blood x 2 (take 3 only if infective endocarditis suspected)

- urine

- if woman has travelled abroad recently or enteric infections suspected, faeces

- if any hint of meningitis, CSF (omit if woman confused or intracranial pressure raised)

- If infection suspected during labour or delivery (e.g. pyrexia, offensive smelling liquor, smelly baby, unexpectedly flat baby at birth), take swabs from vagina, placenta and baby (ear, throat, skin) for microbiology

- Send placenta to histology

Severe sepsis

Add

- If severe sepsis suspected, measure venous plasma lactate

- Arterial blood gases (ABG), acid-base and lactate

- Chest X-ray

- If source of infection not apparent, consider CT scan, ultrasound scan and nuclear medicine imaging

- If woman known to be positive for **ESBL or MGNB**, re-screen for carriage of multi-resistant Gram-negative bacilli with rectal swab and, if urinary catheter *in situ,* CSU

Differential diagnosis

- Systemic disease: occult haemorrhage, myocardial infarction, adrenal insufficiency, pulmonary embolism

OBSERVATIONS

Take and record [on high dependency chart or maternity early warning scoring (MEWS) chart if available locally]

- Temperature

- Heart rate

- Blood pressure using automated non-invasive blood pressure device

- Respiratory rate

- Oxygen saturation

Issue 3
Issued: April 2015
Expires: April 2017

- Peripheral perfusion
- Urinalysis
- Hourly urine output
- Fluid intake, oral and IV
- Lochia if appropriate

Severe sepsis

Observations listed above **plus**

- Level of consciousness, use Glasgow coma scale
- Commence 3 Lead ECG
- If central line inserted, central venous pressure (CVP)
- If gestation appropriate and not delivered, continuous electronic fetal monitoring (EFM)

MANAGEMENT OF PYREXIA IN LABOUR

- If maternal temperature >37.5°C on one occasion:
- keep woman cool
- administer paracetamol 1 g oral repeated 6-hrly as required
- avoid dehydration
- record temperature hourly until apyrexial
- note: temperature rises with epidural *in situ*

High or prolonged pyrexia

- If maternal temperature >38°C once or >37.5°C on two occasions 2 hr apart:
- commence external EFM
- MSU or catheter specimen of urine
- high vaginal swab or low vaginal swab
- blood culture x 2
- Liaise with neonatologists to consider their presence at delivery
- Start IV antibiotics

MANAGEMENT OF SEVERE SEPSIS

Severe sepsis is an emergency. Involve consultant obstetrician at an early stage.

Consultant obstetrician will seek advice from other specialists e.g. anaesthetist, haematologist, microbiologist and intensivist

Key actions (from 'Surviving sepsis')

Tests	Treatment
● FBC and blood cultures before antibiotics ● Measure serum lactate ● Measure urine output hourly	● Broad spectrum antibiotics ● IV fluids ● Oxygen

Airway and breathing

- Adequate oxygen therapy to maintain SpO_2 94–98%
- If increased difficulty in breathing, contact, critical care team to consider intubation and ventilation

Circulation

- Secure IV access with two large bore cannulae
- Avoid siting epidural or spinal anaesthesia
- Ensure adequate fluid replacement
- 20 mL/kg colloid or 40 mL/kg crystalloid [compound sodium lactate (Hartmann's) or sodium chloride 0.9%] over <30 min then reassess
- If no response to simple resuscitation measures, insert CVP line and monitor to guide further fluid replacement
- If anaemic, transfuse blood
- If woman remains hypotensive despite adequate fluid replacement, transfer to critical care for further management

Antibiotics

> *After obtaining urgent bloods, swabs and cultures, administer high dose broad spectrum IV antibiotics immediately without waiting for microbiology results*

- Choice of antibiotic therapy depends on clinical suspicions and local flora and culture information (if available)

- Treatment should include cover for:

- Gram negative and anaerobic organism

- if likelihood of infection is high, Gram-positive cover

- Remove source of infection

- closed-space infections need surgical drainage including evacuation of retained products of conception

- Consider VTE prophylaxis

- Consider delivery

FURTHER MANAGEMENT

- If woman already extremely ill, deteriorates or does not improve, consider additional or alternative IV antibiotics – seek further **early** advice from consultant microbiologist

- repeat microbiological specimens and mark 'urgent'

- In women with endometritis not responding to antibiotics, consider septic pelvic thrombosis

- In presence of uterine sepsis, carefully counsel women requesting conservative management about maternal risks

- Necrotising fasciitis requires early surgical intervention with fasciotomy and aggressive antibiotic therapy

- If Group A *streptococcus* disease suspected, inform neonatologists. If confirmed, this is a notifiable disease.

- Be prepared for haemorrhage from uterine atony and DIC

Issue 3
Issued: April 2015
Expires: April 2017

Sepsis/severe sepsis screening and management flowchart

Does woman have two of the following signs of infection?

- Temperature >38°C or <36°C
- Heart rate:
- >100 bpm (antenatal and intrapartum)
- >90 bpm (postnatal)
- Respiratory rate >20 bpm
- Acutely altered mental state
- WCC >12 OR <4 X 10^9/L (higher threshold in labour)
- Hyperglycaemia (blood glucose >7.7) in the absence of diabetes

Yes

Elicit history or signs of new infection or infective source and consult appropriate guideline

- Prolonged ruptured membranes or offensive smelling liquor
- Unexplained fetal tachycardia in the absence of a maternal tachycardia
- Recent delivery/offensive lochia
- Catheter or dysuria
- Line infection
- Headache with neck stiffness
- Endocarditis
- Breast redness and/or tenderness
- Fetal demise
- Sore throat/cough/sputum/chest pain
- Abdominal pain/distension/diarrhoea
- Cellulitis/wound infection/septic arthritis
- Other

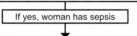
If yes, woman has sepsis

Does woman have signs of organ dysfunction?

- Systolic blood pressure <90 or mean arterial pressure <70 mmHg
- Urine output <0.5 mL/kg/hr for 2 hr
- Platelets <100 x 10^9/L
- Creatinine rise of >44.2 mmol/L or level of >177 mmol/L
- Lactate >2 mmol/L
- New need for oxygen to maintain SpO_2 >90%
- INR >1.5 or PTT >60s
- Bilirubin >70 µmol/L

No   Yes

Treat for sepsis

- Blood cultures
- Lactate
- Fluid balance and catheterise
- Oxygen
- IV antibiotics
- Fluid therapy
- Consider VTE prophylaxis

Woman has severe sepsis

- Start the clock
- Refer to Critical Care
- Administer IV antibiotics within 1 hour – start with stat dose
- Consider operative intervention

DEFINITIONS

- **Pre-eclampsia:** pregnancy induced hypertension with significant proteinuria +/- oedema affecting virtually any organ system in the body
- **Severe pre-eclampsia:** diastolic blood pressure >110 mmHg or systolic blood pressure ≥160 mmHg on more than two occasions, with significant proteinuria
- **Mild to moderate pre-eclampsia:** BP <160/110 and proteinuria with one or more of symptoms and signs listed below (See **RECOGNITION AND ASSESSMENT** below)

Maternal and fetal complications associated with severe pre-eclampsia

Maternal	Fetal
● Eclampsia	● Prematurity
● Placental abruption	● Intrauterine growth restriction
● Severe hypertension	● Acute fetal distress
● Risk of cerebral haemorrhage	● Placental abruption
● Pulmonary oedema	● Intrauterine death
● Renal failure	● Respiratory distress syndrome
● Liver failure or ruptured liver	
● Disseminated intravascular coagulation (DIC)	
● HELLP syndrome	
● Pulmonary haemorrhage	
● Aspiration pneumonia	
● Retinal detachment	
● Circulatory collapse	
● Maternal death	

RECOGNITION AND ASSESSMENT

Symptoms

- Headache
- Visual disturbance
- Epigastric pain
- Vomiting
- Sudden swelling of face, hands or feet
- Oedema

Signs

- Hyperreflexia with clonus
- Abdominal tenderness – right upper quadrant
- Proteinuria of at least 1+ or protein/creatinine ratio of >30 mg/mmol or >0.3 g in 24 hr
- Papilloedema
- Liver tenderness
- Platelet count falling or <100 x 10⁹/L
- Abnormal liver enzymes (ALT or AST rising or >70 IU/L)

Investigations

Urine

- Dipstick measurement; proteinuria of at least 1+
- Confirm significant proteinuria with or without symptoms if:
- ≥300 mg protein in validated 24 hr urine collection or
- urinary protein/creatinine ratio >30 mg/mmol

Issue 3
Issued: April 2015
Expires: April 2017

Blood

- FBC
- If platelet count <100 x 10⁹/L, perform clotting studies
- LFT
- U&E and uric acid
- Group and save

IMMEDIATE MANAGEMENT

- Admit all women with severe pre-eclampsia or eclampsia
- Give high dependency care – see **High dependency care** guideline
- Carefully explain problem and management to woman and birth partner

Multi-disciplinary team planning

- Ensure early involvement and liaison between senior obstetrician, intensive care specialists, delivery suite midwife co-ordinator and neonatologist in assessment and management of women with suspected or proven severe pre-eclampsia and eclampsia

Monitoring

- If in labour, start high dependency care chart in addition to partogram

Minimum requirement

- Maternal pulse and BP – with woman rested and sitting at a 45° angle every 15 min until stabilised, then every 30 min
- ensure appropriate cuff size used and placed at level of heart
- use multiple readings to confirm diagnosis
- use an automated machine that has been validated for use in pregnancy
- Oxygen saturations continually and recorded hourly – obstetric review if <95%
- Respiratory rate hourly
- Fetal heart rate – continually by electronic fetal monitoring (EFM) – see **Electronic fetal monitoring** guideline

Examine

- Optic fundii for signs of haemorrhage and papilloedema
- Assess for hyperreflexia and clonus

TREATMENT

- Give antacid prophylaxis e.g. ranitidine 150 mg oral 6-hrly (if oral inappropriate, 50 mg IM 6-hrly)
- If fetus <35 weeks' gestation, give betamethasone two 12 mg doses IM 12 or 24 hr apart (depending on clinical situation) to promote fetal lung maturity

Blood pressure control

> *The aim of anti-hypertensive therapy is to maintain systolic BP <150 mmHg and prevent cerebral haemorrhage and hypertensive encephalopathy*

When

- In women with a systolic blood pressure >160 mmHg or diastolic blood pressure >110 mmHg, begin antihypertensive treatment

How

- Oral and IV labetalol, oral nifedipine (unlicensed) and IV hydralazine are commonly used agents of choice for severe hypertension – see **Drug treatment regimen** overleaf

Notes

- Consider insertion of arterial line in woman who will be receiving continuous IV antihypertensive; close liaison with anaesthetist is essential
- Consider giving up to 500 mL crystalloid fluid before or at the same time as the first dose of IV hydralazine in the antenatal period
- Avoid rapid fall in blood pressure as this can potentiate fetal distress
- Aim to keep blood pressure <150/80–100 mmHg

Prevention of seizures

- Administer magnesium sulphate prophylaxis – See **Magnesium sulphate** overleaf

Fluid management

Amount of fluid

- Unless there is ongoing haemorrhage, avoid fluid overload – limit total IV input to 1 mL/kg/hr
- include **all** drugs administered in the hourly volume input of fluid
- if oxytocin required, use a reduced fluid oxytocin regimen
- Always use syringe driver or infusion pump to control delivery of fluids

Type of fluid

- If marked hypovolaemia due to haemorrhage (>500 mL), haemolysis or DIC, give blood +/- blood products – discuss with haematologist

Monitoring

- Measure fluid input and output hourly via urinometer
- insert Foley indwelling catheter to measure urine output
- When pre-eclampsia is complicated by pulmonary oedema, persistent oliguria or significant blood loss, consider CVP monitoring after discussion with anaesthetist

Oliguria

- During labour and after delivery, oliguria is not uncommon
- renal failure is unusual in pre-eclampsia and is usually associated with additional problems e.g. haemorrhage and sepsis
- give woman with severe pre-eclampsia controlled fluid and wait for natural diuresis to occur approximately 36–48 hr after delivery
- If oliguria <100 mL over 2 consecutive 4 hr periods, auscultate chest and check U&E, platelet and LFT urgently

- Senior obstetrician or consultant review
- if no signs of fluid overload, give 250 mL colloid fluid challenge and assess response
- if oliguria persists (<50 mL over 4 hr), senior review and consider furosemide and central venous pressure (CVP) monitoring
- if prolonged antenatal oliguria or anuria, prepare for delivery

Thromboembolism

- Give thromboprophylaxis (See **VTE – Thromboprophylaxis** guideline)

DELIVERY

Timing of delivery

- Once woman stable, consultant obstetrician and anaesthetist make decision to deliver. Liaise with neonatology team
- If fetus premature and delivery can be delayed, give betamethasone – two 12 mg doses IM 12 or 24 hr apart (depending on clinical situation) to promote fetal lung maturity. Reassess benefits of continuing the pregnancy after 24 hr

Mode of delivery

- Consider fetal presentation and condition, together with likelihood of success of induction of labour
- after 34 weeks' gestation with a cephalic presentation, consider vaginal delivery
- in <32 weeks' gestation, prefer caesarean section
- If vaginal delivery planned, plan short second stage with consideration of elective operative vaginal delivery

Notes

- An epidural is a useful method of controlling blood pressure and providing analgesia but may be contraindicated in low platelet count
- If oxytocin indicated for induction of labour or augmentation, give IV via a syringe driver and administer a reduced fluid regime

Issue 3
Issued: April 2015
Expires: April 2017

Managing third stage of labour

- Manage third stage with 10 units oxytocin IM (unlicensed) or 5 units IV

> **Do not give ergometrine or syntometrine in any form for prevention of haemorrhage as this can further increase blood pressure**

ECLAMPSIA

- One or more convulsions superimposed on pre-eclampsia
- See **Eclampsia** guideline

HELLP SYNDROME

- Haemolysis, elevated liver enzymes and low platelets (HELLP) occurs in approximately 4–12% of women with severe pre-eclampsia. It is associated with high perinatal mortality

Symptoms

- Can present with vague symptoms which often delay diagnosis
- nausea
- vomiting
- epigastric pain and right upper-quadrant pain
- A unique feature of HELLP syndrome is 'coca-cola' appearance of urine; small amounts of dark black urine are produced

Diagnosis

- Confirmed by:
- fragmented red cells on blood film
- platelet count <100 x 10^9/L
- Elevated AST >75 IU/L significant and >150 IU/L is associated with maternal morbidity
- Severe hypertension is not always a feature of HELLP syndrome and degree of severity rarely reflects overall severity of the disease

Management

As for severe pre-eclampsia plus:
- Evaluate severity

- Hourly BM
- Monitor conscious level and look for signs of confusion
- Stabilise
- Do not use betamethasone or dexamethasone to treat HELLP syndrome
- Early blood transfusion – these women are often profoundly anaemic
- Contact haematologist early for advice about replacement of clotting factors
- **Deliver**
- Postnatal recovery often more complicated, with oliguria and a slow recovery of biochemical parameters

POSTNATAL MANAGEMENT AND FOLLOW-UP

- Up to 44% of convulsions occur postpartum especially at term. Assess carefully and continue high dependency care for a minimum of 24 hr
- Continue antihypertensive medication after delivery
- If BP falls to <130/80 mmHg, reduce antihypertensive treatment
- **While in-patient** – measure BP at least 4 times per day
- **If transferred to community** – measure BP every 1–2 days for up to 2 weeks, until antihypertensive treatment stopped and no hypertension. Medical team to include management plan for monitoring on discharge documentation
- Persisting hypertension and proteinuria at 6 weeks can indicate renal disease, investigate further
- Be aware of risk of late seizures and review carefully before discharge
- Offer follow-up to discuss events, treatment and future pregnancy care
- **Follow-up at 6 weeks**
- Discuss events, treatment and future pregnancy care
- Check BP and urine. Investigate persisting hypertension and proteinuria at 6 weeks as may indicate renal disease, investigate further

DRUG TREATMENT REGIMENS

LABETALOL

- Beta-blocker with additional arteriolar vasodilating action

Common contraindications (see also current BNF)

- Asthma
- Cardiogenic shock
- AV block

Cautions

- Heart failure
- Diabetes

Side effects

- Postural hypotension
- Tiredness
- Headache
- Weakness
- Rashes
- Tingling scalp
- Difficult micturation
- Epigastric pain
- Nausea, vomiting

Labetalol regime on delivery suite

Oral therapy	Acute treatment (IV)	Maintenance treatment (IV)

• If tolerated, 200 mg stat with further 200 mg after 1 hr	• 50 mg IV bolus over 1 min (10 mL labetalol 5 mg/mL)
	• Can be repeated every 5 min to a **maximum** of 200 mg
	• Can cause excessive bradycardia reversed by giving atropine sulphate 600 microgram IV
		• Where continuous IV doses required, consider insertion of arterial line in discussion with anaesthetist
		• Neat labetalol 5 mg/mL at a rate of 4 mL/hr via syringe driver
		• Set target BP and record
		• Start infusion at 4 mL/hr and double every 30 min to maximum 32 mL/hr (150 mg) until BP lowered and stabilised at acceptable level
		• Start at:
		  • 4 mL/hr (double every 30 min if necessary)
		  • 8 mL/hr
		  • 16 mL/hr
		  • 32 mL/hr (maximum)
		
		• Convert to oral therapy – dose dependent on IV dose that was required

Issue 3
Issued: April 2015
Expires: April 2017

NIFEDIPINE

- Calcium-channel blocker, relaxes vascular smooth muscle and dilates coronary and peripheral arteries

Contraindications

- Known hypersensitivity
- Gastrointestinal obstruction
- Hepatic impairment
- Inflammatory bowel disease
- Crohn's disease
- Cardiogenic shock

> **Concurrent use of magnesium sulphate and nifedipine may cause a precipitous drop in blood pressure**

Treatment

- Pre-load with 300 mL of IV colloid before administration
- 10 mg capsule orally, repeat every 30 min, up to 3 doses – Consider SR tablets for longer-term regulation of BP

> **Nifedipine must be swallowed whole – Do not give sublingually**

- Monitor fetal heart rate by continuous electronic fetal monitoring (EFM) – see **Electronic fetal monitoring** guideline
- Measure maternal BP every 5 min in first 30 min after initial administration as may reduce quickly

Side effects

- Headache
- Flushing
- Dizziness
- Tachycardia
- Palpitation
- May induce exaggerated fall in blood pressure

HYDRALAZINE

- Direct acting vasodilator

Contraindications

- Known hypersensitivity
- Idiopathic systemic lupus erythematosus
- Severe tachycardia
- High output heart failure
- Myocardial insufficiency due to mechanical obstruction
- Cor pulmonale
- Dissecting aortic aneurysm
- Acute porphyria

Cautions

- Renal impairment
- Hepatic impairment
- Ischaemic heart disease
- Cerebrovascular disease

Side effects

- Tachycardia
- Palpitations
- Flushing
- Hypotension
- Fluid retention
- Gastrointestinal disturbances
- Headache
- Dizziness
- Rarely: rashes, fever, peripheral neuritis, polyneuritis, paraesthesia, abnormal liver function, agitation, anxiety, dyspnoea

Issue 3
Issued: April 2015
Expires: April 2017

Hydralazine regimen

Acute treatment	Maintenance treatment
● Consider pre-loading with 300 mL colloid before administration	● Where continuous IV doses required, consider insertion of arterial line in discussion with anaesthetist
● 5 mg by slow IV bolus diluted with 10 mL sodium chloride 0.9% – can be repeated after 20–30 min – Some Trusts prefer to mix 20 mg in 20 mL	● 40 mg in 40 mL sodium chloride 0.9% via syringe driver e.g. 1000 microgram/mL solution
● Check BP every 5 min for 30 min or until stable at acceptable limit, then every 15 min for further 60 min	● Start infusion at 2 mL/hr
	● Increase rate in 2 mL/hr increments to a **maximum** of 20 mL/hr
● Continually monitor fetal heart rate by EFM	● If pulse >140, consider alternative hypertensive drug
	● If target BP reached, reduce infusion rate

MAGNESIUM SULPHATE 50%

Cautions

● Renal impairment

● Hepatic impairment

Side effects (generally associated with hypermagnesaemia)

● Nausea

● Vomiting

● Thirst

● Flushing of skin

● Loss of tendon reflexes

● Muscle weakness

● Hypotension

● Arrhythmias

● Respiratory depression

● Drowsiness

● Confusion

● Coma

Seizure prophylaxis

● Administer 2 concentrations:

　● one as loading dose

　● one as continuous infusion for 24 hr or until 24 hr after delivery (or after last seizure or until diuresis, whichever is later)

　● can just be stopped without tapering dose

Magnesium sulphate 50% regimen

Loading dose	Maintenance dose	Dose for recurrent seizures
● 4 g IV ● Add 8 mL (4 g) magnesium sulphate 50% to 12 mL sodium chloride 0.9% – total volume 20 mL ● Administer via syringe driver over 10–20 min (infusion rate of 60–120 mL/hr)	● 1 g/hr IV ● Add 10 mL (5 g) magnesium sulphate 50% to 40 mL sodium chloride 0.9% – total volume 50 mL ● 10 mL = 1 g magnesium sulphate ● Start IV infusion via syringe driver at 10 mL/hr	● Give 2 g bolus for weight <70 kg ● Add 4 mL (2 g) magnesium sulphate 50% to 12 mL sodium chloride 0.9% and administer by slow bolus injection over 5–10 min ● Give 4 g bolus for weight >70 kg ● Add 8 mL (4 g) magnesium sulphate 50% to 12 mL sodium chloride 0.9% and administer by slow bolus injection over 5–10 min ● Increase maintenance dose to 2 g/hr IV

Observations

- Continuous pulse oximetry
- Urine output hourly
- Respiratory rate hourly
- Deep tendon reflexes

Check serum magnesium levels

Stop magnesium sulphate if:

- Urine output <100 mL in 4 hr
- Respiratory rate ≤12 breaths/min
- Oxygen saturation <90%
- Patellar reflexes absent (not due to regional anaesthesia)

97% of magnesium is excreted in urine. Oliguria can lead to toxicity.

Antidote – 10 mL calcium gluconate 10% IV over 10 min

DEFINITION

Prolonged head to body delivery time (>60 sec) requiring additional obstetric manoeuvres to release shoulders from behind mother's pubic bone

RISK FACTORS

- It is advisable for middle grade obstetrician (ST3–7 or equivalent e.g. staff grade, clinical fellow) to be on delivery suite or in the delivery room dependent on the level of risk. This tends to be women with previous shoulder dystocia

Antepartum

Maternal

- Maternal obesity – body mass index >30 kg/m^2 (see **Obese mother** guideline)
- Excessive weight gain
- Previous big baby
- Previous shoulder dystocia
- Maternal diabetes mellitus – even in absence of fetal macrosmia

Fetal

- Suspected or confirmed fetal macrosmia
- Post-dated pregnancy

Intrapartum

- Labour abnormalities e.g. mid-pelvic operative vaginal deliveries
- Prolonged first or second stage
- Oxytocic augmentation
- Poor descent of fetal head
- Assisted delivery
- Signs in second stage:
- difficulty with delivery of the face and chin
- the head remaining tightly applied to the vulva or even retracting (turtle-neck sign)
- failure of restitution of the fetal head
- failure of the shoulders to descend

> *If any of the above are identified, notify middle grade obstetrician and request presence on delivery suite*

MANAGEMENT

Immediate action

- Sound emergency call bell or buzzer and summon:
- senior midwife
- senior obstetrician
- neonatal team member (as per local practice)
- Quickly tell mother what is happening, reassure her
- Nominate a member of staff to document events
- If time allows:
- anaesthetist
- theatre staff

Position woman and traction

- Position mother with buttocks at end of bed lying flat
- Mother's legs flexed, abducted and rotated outwards (McRoberts manoeuvre) and attempt delivery using routine axial traction

> *To reduce risk of brachial plexus injury, use axial traction only*

- Quickly remove end of bed

Suprapubic pressure

- If delivery not successful, ask assistant to apply suprapubic pressure for 30 sec with heel of hand over posterior aspect of shoulder – **assistant must be aware of position of fetal back to ensure pressure applied in the right direction**
- if continuous pressure not successful, attempt a rocking movement
- if shoulder becomes disimpacted, encourage mother to push and attempt delivery

Issue 3
Issued: April 2015
Expires: April 2017

Subsequent management

- If delivery unsuccessful, performing clinician should attempt either of the 2 manoeuvres **below** independently to attempt rotation of the shoulders
- base decision on which manoeuvre to use first, on training and clinical expertise, and the clinical circumstances
- if first fails try second manoeuvre
- Perform episiotomy to facilitate access

Delivery of posterior arm

- Attempt delivery of posterior arm and shoulder:
- pass a hand to reach fetal axilla and hook shoulder down bringing posterior arm within reach
- deliver posterior arm by performing backward pressure on the cubital fossa
- grasp hand and sweep across chest and face leading to subsequent delivery of shoulder and body

Wood's screw/Rubin II manoeuvre

- Insert hand into vagina and approach posterior shoulder from **front** of fetus, aiming to rotate shoulder towards symphysis pubis
- Insert fingers of opposite hand **behind** anterior shoulder pushing shoulder towards the chest
- combination of these two manoeuvres frees the impacted shoulders and allows delivery
- If unsuccessful, consider reverse Wood's screw manoeuvre

Reverse Wood's screw

- Insert hand into vagina and approach posterior shoulder from **behind** the fetus in an attempt to rotate in opposite direction to the original Woods Screw. If successful, the shoulders will rotate 180 degrees in the opposite direction and deliver

Above actions unsuccessful

- Position mother on all-fours (Gaskin manoeuvre) and attempt delivery of posterior shoulder repeating above manoeuvres
- When all above manoeuvres have been attempted, choose either the Zavenelli manoeuvre or symphysiotomy

Zavenelli manoeuvre

- A consultant or senior obstetrician may use the Zavenelli manoeuvre: rotation, flexion and reinsertion of fetal head into vagina, followed by emergency caesarean section

Symphysiotomy

- Syphysiotomy can be used **as a last resort** and only by, or in the presence of consultant obstetrician
- insert a urethral catheter to move urethra to one side, make a midline incision in symphyseal joint and perform delivery
- to avoid sudden abduction, ensure mother's legs are supported at all times

AFTER DELIVERY

- Hand baby to waiting neonatal team member who will perform resuscitation where required – see **Cardiopulmonary resuscitation of the newborn** guideline
- Delivering midwife/medical staff will perform active management of the third stage
- inspect genital tract thoroughly and repair
- Ensure adequate analgesia, antibiotics and/or laxatives prescribed
- Perform maternal observations and estimation of blood loss
- In all cases of shoulder dystocia, obtain paired cord blood for gases – see **Umbilical cord sampling** guideline

Documentation

- In all cases of shoulder dystocia, regardless of outcome, midwife or doctor responsible for mother's care should:

- complete a shoulder dystocia checklist and place one copy in maternal healthcare record

- record which shoulder was anterior at delivery

- follow local adverse incident/near miss reporting procedure

Communication with parents/family

- Obstetrician and midwife must discuss events with woman/family and document discussion in maternal healthcare record

- If baby well, encourage a period of skin-to-skin contact

Examination of baby

- Neonatal team member who was present at delivery will carry out a detailed initial examination – see Staffordshire, Shropshire & Black Country Newborn and Maternity Network **Examination of the newborn** guideline (if used locally), paying particular attention to the arms for the presence of swelling, bruising, tone, posture and movement. If there are concerns, X-ray of affected side – arm and clavicle

- **No movement noted** – inform neonatal consultant on duty and refer to surgeons for review and investigation of possible brachial plexus injury – see Staffordshire, Shropshire & Black Country Newborn and Maternity Network **Upper limb birth injuries** guideline

- **Some restricted movement noted** – refer to physiotherapy and arrange out-patient follow-up

- **Baby appears well** – transfer to postnatal ward with mother. A full neonatal assessment will take place, and findings documented in maternal healthcare record, before discharge from hospital

Transfer to postnatal ward

- When transferring mother and baby to postnatal ward, follow local practice and ensure all events communicated to postnatal ward midwives

- Obstetrician involved in the shoulder dystocia will:

- visit woman and family on postnatal ward the following day to discuss events in detail

- if appropriate speak to other healthcare professionals involved e.g. neonatologist or midwife

Deterioration in baby's condition

- If, at any time, midwifery staff in hospital or community detect deterioration in baby's condition, refer to neonatal team

In hospital

- Contact neonatal junior doctor and/or middle grade depending on severity of problem

In the community

- Contact woman's GP/Paediatric Assessment Unit or A&E department depending on severity of problem

- For babies with a history of shoulder dystocia, follow local incident reporting policy for re-admission

DISCHARGE AND FOLLOW-UP

- Neonatal staff will discuss ongoing care with parents/family before discharge

Algorithm: Management of shoulder dystocia (MOET course manual 2007)

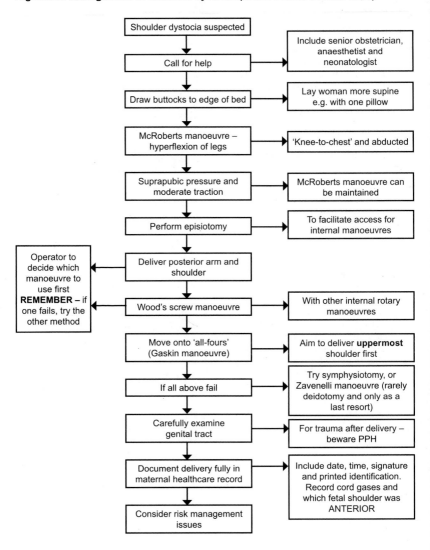

Shoulder dystocia suspected
↓
Call for help → Include senior obstetrician, anaesthetist and neonatologist
↓
Draw buttocks to edge of bed → Lay woman more supine e.g. with one pillow
↓
McRoberts manoeuvre – hyperflexion of legs → 'Knee-to-chest' and abducted
↓
Suprapubic pressure and moderate traction → McRoberts manoeuvre can be maintained
↓
Perform episiotomy → To facilitate access for internal manoeuvres
↓
Deliver posterior arm and shoulder ← Operator to decide which manoeuvre to use first **REMEMBER** – if one fails, try the other method
↓
Wood's screw manoeuvre → With other internal rotary manoeuvres
↓
Move onto 'all-fours' (Gaskin manoeuvre) → Aim to deliver **uppermost** shoulder first
↓
If all above fail → Try symphysiotomy, or Zavenelli manoeuvre (rarely deidotomy and only as a last resort)
↓
Carefully examine genital tract → For trauma after delivery – beware PPH
↓
Document delivery fully in maternal healthcare record → Include date, time, signature and printed identification. Record cord gases and which fetal shoulder was ANTERIOR
↓
Consider risk management issues

INTRODUCTION

- Some Trusts do not support commercial stem cell collection

- If your Trust is not licensed for the collection of cord blood, collection for commercial or non-commercial reasons must be performed under a third party agreement with a Human Tissue Authority licensed establishment

- The professional collecting cord blood must be appropriately trained to ensure an uncontaminated sample that is safe to use

- Fetal wellbeing takes priority. If compromised for any reason, stem cell collection will be delayed or, in some circumstances, not possible

- Umbilical cord collection must not interfere with the care of mother or baby

- Do not delay mother and baby skin-to-skin contact

> *If a family wishes to undergo umbilical cord blood collection, discussion must take place as early in the antenatal period as possible to allow time for necessary arrangements*

- Cord blood collection is particularly unlikely to be possible in the following circumstances:

- prematurity

- nuchal cord

- multiple pregnancy

- emergency caesarean section

- postpartum haemorrhage

COMMERCIAL BLOOD COLLECTION

- If woman is interested in commercial cord blood collection, advise her that collection for commercial storage is not permitted on most NHS Trust premises unless there is a private arrangement with a company licenced under Regulation 7 (1) and Schedule 2 of Human Tissue (quality and safety for human application) Regulations 2007

- Woman is responsible for this private arrangement. She will inform her community midwife of her plan

- Community midwife or other maternity professional will inform midwifery manager according to local protocols and document in maternal healthcare record

- The company (e.g. 'Cells 4 life') will confirm the plan in writing for the woman. File this in the maternal healthcare record

- Woman's birth partner will contact the private phlebotomist to arrange stem cell collection following birth

- Midwives or doctors must never, in any circumstances, be involved in the collection of cord blood for commercial stem cell storage

- The company accepts liability for failed sample. Therefore, the Trust does not have legal responsibility or liability for samples taken on their premises

Issue 3
Issued: April 2015
Expires: April 2017

NON-COMMERCIAL BLOOD COLLECTION

- Umbilical cord blood may be collected via a third party agreement with a Human Tissue Authority licensed establishment. Collection may have been recommended where family members have:

- haemoglobinopathies

- acute inherited disorders

- acute lymphoblastic leukaemia

- In general, those caring for the family member with the haematological disorder have provided third party agreement for cord blood collection. They also have the responsibility to provide training and clear instructions for staff

- The National Blood Service in Birmingham (if involved) provides two collection packs containing instructions and contact details. One pack is for staff (most likely to be present when collection occurs) to open and familiarise themselves with before delivery. **Do not open** the second pack until cord blood collection is about to be performed

- Store the cool packs in a refrigerator at 4°C until required – **Do not freeze**

- In addition to the collection packs, ensure the following equipment is available:

- Spencer-Wells clamps

- scissors

- swabs, spray and gauze for cord disinfection before venepuncture

Collection

- See NHS Blood and Transplant Service http://www.nhsbt.nhs.uk/

INTRODUCTION

Maternal drug use in pregnancy can seriously affect fetal growth. When multiple drugs are taken against a background of other adverse social conditions, (poor nutrition, smoking and alcohol use), fetal outcome can be very poor

Many drugs (opiates, benzodiazepines) can cause severe neonatal withdrawal symptoms

Substance misuse can lead to poor maternal health e.g. infective endocarditis, VTE and blood borne viruses

Every maternity unit should provide an accessible and non-judgmental service for pregnant problem drug users, and should be able to offer high quality care aimed at minimising the impact of the mother's drug use on the pregnancy and the baby

Ensure social care is in place before baby is discharged

ANTENATAL CARE

- Initial contact between woman and maternity services is likely to influence their subsequent uptake of care. Non-judgmental care from maternity unit staff encourages regular attendance, which in turn improves antenatal care, detection of fetal growth restriction, neonatal care, communication between members of the multiagency team, and discharge planning
- Whilst respecting privacy and confidentiality, routinely record problem drug or alcohol use at booking risk assessment

Booking

- For women who disclose substance misuse:
- book under consultant care to facilitate planning of maternity, neonatal and social care within a multidisciplinary team
- inform specialist midwife

Specialist midwife/drug worker will

- Discuss neonatal abstinence syndrome and plan of care with woman and appropriate family members
- Initiate child safeguarding procedure
- Encourage women using opiates who are not already in a drug treatment programme, to accept referral to specialist services for:
- a full assessment of substance usage
- drug screening (to confirm present usage)
- ongoing counselling
- support in stabilising usage through substitute prescribing (e.g. methadone)
- thorough assessment of woman's social circumstances to decide appropriate referral (e.g. social care and health planning)
- Record and discuss with community midwife
- Refer woman to appropriate professionals

Neonatal alert

- Initiate neonatal alert process in line with local practice

Documentation and confidentiality

- Be aware – although the maternal hand-held record is marked 'confidential', anything written can be read by others. Before recording explicit details of substance misuse in this record, ensure woman agrees to their inclusion

Issue 3
Issued: April 2015
Expires: April 2017

Domestic abuse

- Staff should be aware that substance misuse may be associated with current or past experiences of abuse. Domestic abuse often escalates during pregnancy
- As a minimum, ensure routine enquiries about domestic abuse are made at booking
- Whenever possible, woman should be seen alone at least once during the antenatal period to enable disclosure more easily

Screening for blood-borne viruses

- In addition to routine Hepatitis B and HIV screening, advise routine Hepatitis C screening

Hepatitis B and C

- See **Hepatitis** guideline

HIV

- See **HIV positive women** guideline

Plan of antenatal care

Gestation	Action
At first disclosure	● Consultant-led antenatal clinic ● Complete CAF form (if used locally) ● Liaise with specialist midwife

Booking	● Find out which substances are being used and in what quantities
	● Arrange following tests:
	  booking bloods
	  Hepatitis C
	  dating scan
	● Discuss serum screening for Down's syndrome
	● Ensure follow-up with specialist drug workers
	● Plan subsequent antenatal visits with community midwife/antenatal clinic

18–23 weeks	● Anomaly scan
Third trimester	● Growth scan (according to local policy) ● Repeat bloods ● Ensure pre-birth plan in place, if appropriate ● Review plan of care for baby
41 weeks	● Induction of labour for obstetric reasons

Non-booked women

- On admission, women who have not engaged with maternity services (who deliver within the Trust) require:
- urgent screening for blood-borne viruses
- detailed multi-agency discharge planning
- referral to social services (via CAF form if used locally)

DNAs

- See local protocol for follow-up of women who do not attend scheduled antenatal clinical appointments
- Ensure specialist drug worker or team is informed of woman's failure to attend. They may be able to encourage attendance by engaging with her in a non-hospital setting
- If woman persistently fails to attend booked antenatal clinic appointments, refer to specialist midwife

CANNABIS MISUSE

- Cannabis can be taken orally or smoked with tobacco

Risks

- Smoking tobacco can cause fetal growth restriction, preterm labour, stillbirth and sudden infant death. Encourage smoking cessation

Action

- Follow local policy

ALCOHOL MISUSE

- Consuming alcohol during pregnancy can damage the fetus. Explain the risks and advise woman to avoid alcohol consumption (including binge-drinking in early pregnancy)

Estimating alcohol intake during pregnancy

- Ask woman about alcohol intake during pregnancy, but be aware they often under-report and underestimate their true intake

Action

- If woman is drinking heavily, stopping suddenly may be hazardous to her and the baby – seek specialist advice and referral
- Check booking liver function tests and consider liver scan if markedly abnormal
- Fetal anomaly scan
- Growth scan as local policy
- The use of Antabuse® (disulfiram) is contraindicated in pregnancy and breastfeeding

OPIATE MISUSE

Action

- Encourage woman to enter into an opiate maintenance programme [methadone or buprenorphine (Subutex®)] with drug treatment services who can provide counselling, health promotion and help with social care support
- Consider increasing methadone/Subutex® dose in third trimester (plasma concentrations may decrease as gestation increases). Increase will need to be reversed in the postpartum period (if mother is highly motivated)

BENZODIAZEPINES (DIAZEPAM, TEMAZEPAM) MISUSE

- Benzodiazepine misuse is commonly associated with other substance misuse. It is essential to consider this when formulating an antenatal plan of care
- Maternal benzodiazepine dependence is associated with neonatal abstinence syndrome, sometimes prolonged, but is not associated with any other adverse pregnancy outcomes
- Avoid abrupt withdrawal – sudden withdrawal from benzodiazepines can precipitate severe anxiety, hallucinations and seizures

ADMISSION AND MATERNAL IN-PATIENT CARE

On admission to maternity unit

- For any planned admission, ensure clear plan involving community pharmacy where woman is obtaining opiate replacement therapy
- If admitted as an emergency, consultant obstetrician will decide appropriate opiate replacement dosage (follow local policy to ascertain usual dosage)
- timing of administration of opiate replacement should follow woman's normal pattern
- **Do not** prescribe opiate replacement therapy to take home – arrange supply to be available from woman's usual source

Labour and pain relief

- Inform specialist drug worker/team
- Give usual dose of methadone during labour at the regular time, although this will not be adequate for pain relief in labour
- If woman Subutex® (buprenorphine) user, adequate pain relief can be difficult as it can reduce the effects of opioid analgesics
- Morphine and pethidine may be inadequate for pain relief; regional analgesia may be preferable – involve on-call anaesthetist early
- Standard opiate analgesia can safely be given
- Inform neonatologists when delivery imminent. It is not necessary for them to attend routinely unless there are other indications

> ***DO NOT GIVE naloxone to baby as there is a major risk of respiratory depression and seizures***

POSTNATAL CARE

Neonatal abstinence syndrome

- See Staffordshire, Shropshire & Black Country Newborn and Maternity Network **Abstinence syndrome** guideline (if used locally)

Baby

- Encourage breastfeeding
- Be aware of:
- late neonatal abstinence syndrome (>72 hr)
- benzodiazepines have longer withdrawal period
- Advise mothers of neonatal abstinence syndrome symptoms and signs
- Give contact number for community midwife and provide a means for mother and baby to return if worried (fast track, symptom awareness)
- Arrange community midwife visit
- Arrange follow-up clinic appointment. Duration and frequency of follow-up will be individualised

Mother

- Inform woman's specialist drug worker of discharge
- Multi-professional meeting with social care and health plan
- Ensure prescriptions in place in the community (especially if discharged before a week-end)

CLASSIFICATION

Third degree tear

- Injury to perineum involving the anal sphincter complex:

- 3a: <50% of external anal sphincter (EAS) thickness torn

- 3b: >50% of EAS thickness torn

- 3c: EAS and internal anal sphincter (IAS) torn

Fourth degree tear

- Injury to perineum involving anal sphincter complex (EAS and IAS) and anal epithelium

> *If tear involved anal mucosa only with intact anal sphincter complex (buttonhole tear), document as a separate entity.*
>
> *If not detected and repaired, this type of tear may result in a recto-vaginal fistula*

RISK FACTORS

- Forceps delivery

- Second stage >1 hour

- Shoulder dystocia

- Nulliparity

- Persistent occipitoposterior position

- Midline episiotomy

- Birth weight >4 kg

- Induction of labour

ASSESSMENT OF PERINEAL TRAUMA

- See also **Perineal trauma** guideline

- Systematically examine women who sustain genital tract trauma during vaginal birth to assess severity of damage, include: rectal examination to exclude damage to sphincter complex (external and internal anal sphincters and rectal mucosa)

> *Informed verbal consent must be obtained before performing rectal examination*

- If practitioner inexperienced in assessing perineal damage or unsure of degree of trauma sustained, seek a second opinion

Documentation

- Clearly document in mother's healthcare record:

- examination findings, using agreed classification above

- if rectal examination performed as part of initial assessment before suturing

- if rectal examination was not carried out and reasons for **not** doing so

PRINCIPLES OF REPAIR

> *Obstetric anal sphincter repair to be performed only by an appropriately trained, competent practitioner.*
>
> *Practitioners who have not been assessed as competent must be supervised by an experienced clinician*

Technique and position of woman

> *Use aseptic technique at all stages of procedure*

- Suture as soon as possible following delivery to reduce bleeding and risk of infection

- Obtain written informed consent before undertaking repair

- Perform rectal examination before suturing to assess the integrity of the rectal mucosa and confirm extent of damage

- Perform repair, in theatre, with mother in lithotomy position using good lighting

- Use regional or general anaesthesia (to allow relaxation of the anal sphincter to enable torn ends to be brought together without tension)

- Depending on full extent of injury, perform repair to anal sphincter complex in following sequence

Rectal mucosa

- Use interrupted or continuous sutures with 2–0 Vicryl Rapide or equivalent on round bodied needle

Internal anal sphincter (IAS)

- Use interrupted mattress sutures using 3–0 PDS or equivalent on round bodied needle or 2-0 Polysorb or equivalent on round bodied needle

External anal sphincter (EAS)

- Identify torn ends of the EAS and apply Allis tissue forceps

- Repair using either an overlap or end-to-end approximation technique with either 3/0 PDS round bodied needle or 2–0 Vicryl or equivalent on round bodied needle

- If overlap technique used it may be necessary to dissect the EAS to facilitate this (remember not to over-dissect as this may cause pudendal nerve damage)

Overlap method   End-end method

Vagina, perineal muscles and skin

- Identify apex of vaginal mucosa and place first stitch slightly beyond it

- Repair vaginal wall tissues with a continuous non-locking stitch

- Repair deeper perineal muscles using a continuous suture, closing the skin with a continuous subcutaneous suture using Vicryl Rapide 2/0 material on taper cut needle

- Following completion of repair, carry out rectal examination to ensure sutures **have not** been placed through the rectal mucosa

Analgesia

- Ibuprofen 400 mg oral 8-hrly (check not allergic to NSAID)

- Appropriate non-codeine-based oral analgesia e.g. paracetamol

INTRA-OPERATIVE MANAGEMENT

Antibiotics

- Follow local antibiotics prescribing policy

POST-OPERATIVE MANAGEMENT

- Insert an indwelling Foley catheter and leave *in situ* in accordance with local practice

Laxatives

- Ispaghula husk 3.5 g twice daily for 10 days

- Lactulose 10 mL 8-hrly for 10 days

Oral antibiotics

- Follow local antibiotic prescribing policy

DOCUMENTATION

In cases of obstetric anal sphincter injury, follow local risk management procedure and document in medical record

- The following must be documented:
- classification of injury including anatomical structures involved
- method of repair and suture materials used
- anaesthetic used
- if rectal examination carried out following repair and verbal consent obtained
- estimated blood loss
- instruments, sharps and swabs accounted for, including names of those checking
- whether woman fully informed about the nature of her injury
- appropriate information given to the woman – extent of trauma, diet, perineal hygiene, pelvic floor exercises and follow-up arrangements

DISCHARGE AND FOLLOW-UP

- Give woman instructions on pelvic floor exercises, diet, hygiene and pain relief
- Arrange review appointment at 6 weeks postpartum – If available, in perineal care clinic
- Otherwise, follow local practice
- If available locally, provide patient information leaflet

DEFINITION

Time from birth of baby to expulsion of placenta and membranes and control of bleeding

Information for woman

Inform woman in the antenatal period, that active management of third stage shortens its duration and reduces risk of postpartum haemorrhage (PPH). However, women at low risk of PPH and who request a physiological third stage should be supported in their choice

ACTIVE MANAGEMENT

- Care package including:
- routine use of uterotonic drugs – oxytocin alone (Syntocinon 10 units IM or 5 units by slow IV bolus), or with ergometrine (Syntometrine)
- do not give Syntometrine to a woman who has been hypertensive or whose blood pressure has not been checked since admission
- early clamping and cutting of cord, after at least one minute for a healthy term infant to allow placental fetal transfusion to occur
- controlled cord traction (CCT)

PHYSIOLOGICAL MANAGEMENT

- Care package including:
- no uterotonic drugs
- encourage skin-to-skin contact and early breastfeeding
- no clamping and cutting of cord until pulsation has ceased
- placenta delivered by maternal effort and gravity
- Do not pull cord or palpate uterus
- if delivery of placenta required owing to bleeding or delay or if requested by woman, administer a uterotonic drug as part of active management

> *Third stage is prolonged if not completed within 30 minutes with active management and 60 minutes with physiological management*

OBSERVATIONS

- Observe and record at least once after delivery
- temperature
- pulse
- blood pressure
- respiratory rate

ASSESS

- General physical condition
- Maternal colour
- Uterine tone
- Blood loss
- Is bladder empty? See **Bladder care** guideline
- Emotional/psychological condition

EXAMINE

- When delivered:
- cord
- placenta
- membranes
- perineum – see **Perineal trauma** guideline
- Take umbilical cord blood sample for gases (see **Umbilical cord sampling** guideline) and for haemolytic disease of the newborn (HDN) testing if required

COMPLICATIONS

- In postpartum haemorrhage, emergency action is required – see **Postpartum haemorrhage** guideline
- See also, **Third and fourth degree perineal tears** guideline, **Collapse** guideline and **Retained placenta** guideline

INTRODUCTION

- In randomised clinical trials, transcervical catheter induction has been shown to be safe and effective in inducing labour in women with an unfavourable cervical score

- Its aim is to gradually dilate the cervix by gentle and constant pressure of the catheter balloon at the level of the cervix

> *Transcervical catheter induction is an obstetric consultant decision. Do not use routinely*

INDICATIONS

- Unfavourable cervix requiring induction of labour where artificial rupture of membranes (ARM) is not possible

- Previous caesarean section

- Failed attempt at prostaglandin induction

CONTRAINDICATIONS

- Ruptured membranes

METHOD

Consent

- Discuss procedure with woman and obtain and document verbal consent

Equipment

- Foley balloon catheter 30 mL balloon or Cook's cervical ripening balloon catheter

- both are effective but the Foley catheter is cheaper and has a shorter placement-to-delivery interval

- Instillagel® (local anaesthetic and antiseptic)

- Sterile vaginal examination pack

- Sterile Cusco speculum

- Sponge-holding forceps (Rampley's)

- Entonox

- Antiseptic solution

- 100 mL sterile water or sodium chloride 0.9%

Procedure

- Ensure woman's bladder is empty and transfer to delivery suite

- Insert Instillagel® into vagina 5–10 min before procedure to reduce discomfort when manipulating cervix. Entonox should be available

- Place woman in lithotomy position

- Clean vulva with antiseptic solution

- It may be necessary to gently grasp the anterior cervical lip with sponge-holding forceps to achieve a good view and facilitate procedure. This can be uncomfortable and should not be done routinely

Foley catheter

- Hold (do not clamp) catheter with Rampley's forceps 1–3 cm (i.e. measured cervical length from vaginal examination) from the end of the balloon area

- Advance into the cervical canal until 1–3 cm from the balloon area has entered the canal and inflate the balloon with 30 mL of sterile water or sodium chloride 0.9%

- Gently pull catheter back to ensure balloon is resting at the internal cervical os

- Apply a spigot to the catheter and tape catheter to the thigh under gentle tension

Cook's catheter

- Pass the catheter through the cervix until both balloons have entered the cervix

- Inflate the intrauterine (red) balloon with 40 mL sterile water or sodium chloride 0.9%

- Pull the catheter back until the balloon is against the internal os

- Fill the visible vaginal (green) balloon with 20 mL sterile water or sodium chloride 0.9%

Issue 3
Issued: April 2015
Expires: April 2017

Post-insertion

- Perform electronic fetal monitoring (EFM). See **Electronic fetal monitoring** guideline

- Observe for signs and symptoms of labour, spontaneous expulsion of balloon, ruptured membranes, febrile symptoms, pain and vaginal bleeding

- If catheter has not been passed vaginally (12 hr for Cook's or 18 hr for Foley's), remove

- Senior obstetrician will decide whether ARM is possible. If not, options include a further attempt or caesarean section

All staff involved in maternity care should receive at least annual training in the management of obstetric emergencies including umbilical cord prolapse

DEFINITION

Descent of umbilical cord through cervix alongside (occult) or past presenting part (overt) in the presence of ruptured membranes

Background

- Incidence of cord prolapse is between 0.1–0.6%

- 50% of cases are preceded by obstetric manipulation

- Cord prolapse carries a perinatal mortality rate of 91/1000

- in hospital settings, mortality is largely secondary to prematurity and congenital malformations

- Cord prolapse is also associated with birth asphyxia

- asphyxia, predominantly caused by cord compression and umbilical arterial vasospasm, can result in long-term morbidity because of hypoxic ischaemic encephalopathy

RECOGNITION AND ASSESSMENT

Symptoms and signs

- Cord presentation and prolapse may occur with no outward physical signs and with a normal fetal heart rate pattern

- Abnormal fetal heart rate pattern (e.g. bradycardia, variable decelerations, prolonged deceleration of >1 min – particularly if soon after membrane rupture)

- Cord seen or felt at vaginal examination

Investigations

- Auscultate fetal heart soon after rupture of membranes

- Routine vaginal examination is **not** indicated if liquor clear with spontaneous rupture of membranes in the presence of normal fetal heart rate and absence of risk factors

Cord prolapse suspected

- Suspect where there is an abnormal fetal heart rate pattern (e.g. bradycardia, variable decelerations), particularly if such changes occur soon after membrane rupture, spontaneously or with amniotomy

- Perform speculum and/or digital vaginal examination (even at preterm gestation)

- Do **not** perform ultrasound examination to predict increased probability of cord prolapse

Table 1: Risk factors associated with cord prolapse

General risk factors	Procedure related
● Low birth weight (<2.5 kg) ● Prematurity (<37 wk) ● Fetal congenital anomalies ● Breech presentation ● Transverse, oblique and unstable lie ● Second twin ● Polyhydramnios ● Unengaged presenting part ● Low-lying placenta, other abnormal placentation	● Artificial rupture of membranes ● Vaginal manipulation of fetus with ruptured membranes ● External cephalic version (during procedure) ● Internal podalic version ● Stabilising induction of labour

IMMEDIATE TREATMENT

Follow **Flowchart** and **General principles** below

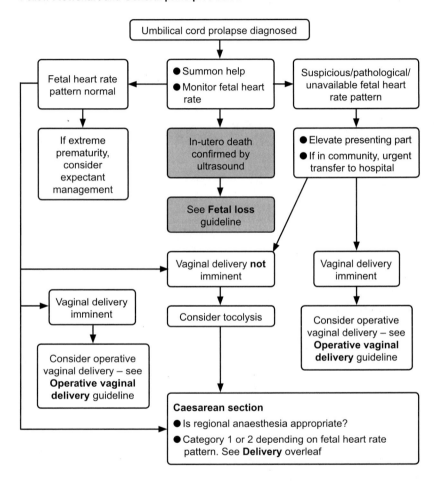

Umbilical cord prolapse diagnosed

- Summon help
- Monitor fetal heart rate

Fetal heart rate pattern normal

Suspicious/pathological/unavailable fetal heart rate pattern

If extreme prematurity, consider expectant management

In-utero death confirmed by ultrasound

See **Fetal loss** guideline

- Elevate presenting part
- If in community, urgent transfer to hospital

Vaginal delivery **not** imminent

Vaginal delivery imminent

Vaginal delivery imminent

Consider tocolysis

Consider operative vaginal delivery – see **Operative vaginal delivery** guideline

Consider operative vaginal delivery – see **Operative vaginal delivery** guideline

Caesarean section
- Is regional anaesthesia appropriate?
- Category 1 or 2 depending on fetal heart rate pattern. See **Delivery** overleaf

General principles

- To prevent vasospasm, minimise handling of loops of cord lying outside vagina
- Manual replacement of prolapsed cord above presenting part is not recommended
- Wrapping cord in swabs soaked in warm sodium chloride 0.9% is of no proven benefit
- Attempt to prevent cord compression by:

Manual elevation of presenting part

Contraindications

- Procedure resulting in unnecessary delay in delivery

Procedure

- Insert gloved hand or 2 fingers into vagina and apply pressure to presenting part pushing it upwards
- Once presenting part above pelvic brim, apply suprapubic pressure upwards

Complications

- Excessive displacement of presenting part may result in more cord prolapsing

Bladder filling to elevate presenting part

Indications

- Decision-to-delivery interval likely to be prolonged and/or involve ambulance transfer

Contraindications

- Procedure resulting in unnecessary delay in delivery

Procedure

- Catheterise woman with appropriate Foley catheter
- Insert end of a blood-giving set into end of Foley catheter and, once 500–750 mL sodium chloride 0.9% instilled, clamp catheter

- Empty bladder just before any delivery attempt
- woman adopting knee-chest position or head-down tilt (preferably in left-lateral position)
- While preparing for caesarean section, consider tocolysis if fetal heart rate abnormalities persist after attempts to prevent compression and when delivery is likely to be delayed
- do not allow above to cause unnecessary delay

Gestational age at the limits of viability

- In cases of cord prolapse complicating pregnancies with gestational age at the limits of viability:
- counsel mother on continuation and termination of pregnancy

Delivery

- When vaginal delivery **not** imminent, caesarean section
- **Category 1** (caesarean section performed with the aim of delivering within ≤30 min) if cord prolapse associated with suspicious or pathological fetal heart rate pattern – providing maternal safety is not unduly compromised
- **Category 2** if fetal heart rate pattern normal
- If vaginal birth imminent, vaginal birth is preferable to caesarean section
- if quick and safe delivery anticipated, attempt vaginal birth (in most cases operative) at full dilatation
- In some circumstances (e.g. internal podalic version for a second twin) breech extraction may be performed
- Cord blood samples for pH and base excess measurement – see **Umbilical cord sampling** guideline

SUBSEQUENT MANAGEMENT

- Offer mother postnatal debriefing
- Local clinical incident procedure for all cases of umbilical cord prolapse

Issue 3
Issued: April 2015
Expires: April 2017

INDICATIONS

May include

- Baby born in poor condition – Apgar score of ≤5 at 1 min
- Suspicious or pathological electronic fetal monitoring (EFM) trace
- Shoulder dystocia
- Instrumental delivery
- Caesarean section – elective (if local practice) and emergency
- Antepartum haemorrhage
- Meconium staining of liquor
- Fetal blood sample is taken during labour
- Premature delivery
- Breech presentation
- Intra-uterine growth retardation (IUGR)
- Insulin dependant diabetes in pregnancy
- Maternal pyrexia in labour
- Cholestasis in pregnancy
- Multiple pregnancy

PROCEDURE

Timing

- Collect samples ideally within 30 min following placental delivery
- blood will not normally clot while still in cord
- sampling within 30 min with cord stored at room temperature and taken with a good technique will provide most reliable results
- If delay of >30 min anticipated, refrigerate section of cord and sample within 1 hour post-delivery

Method

- Once baby separated from placenta, isolate and double clamp section of cord selected for sampling as soon as possible
- Insert needle at 30 degree angle to vessel to ensure sampling from single vessel
- For best results, fill 2 mL pre-heparinised syringe. Ensure all air bubbles expelled
- Obtain sample from both artery and vein

Results

- Occlude syringe with cap following sampling, reducing exposure to air
- Analyse in blood gas analyser
- Secure results in intrapartum notes. As a minimum, document cord pH and base excess in maternal healthcare record

Action

- Inform postnatal ward on transfer of any low pH and high base excess, obtained from blood analysis, even if baby in good condition
- Low cord pH – follow local guidelines for neonatal management following delivery
- Babies born with cord pH levels <7.0 – follow local incident reporting procedure

DEFINITION

Uterine rupture

- Separation of uterine muscle requiring operative intervention or is symptomatic. Involves full thickness of the uterine wall

- uterine rupture is most often seen in women with a scarred uterus (usually from a previous caesarean section)

- uterine rupture can occur in women who have not had uterine surgery

Dehiscence

- Scar starts to separate, but mother and baby are not affected. No symptoms are evident. Dehiscence is noted at repeat caesarean section

True uterine rupture

- Symptomatic causing fetal distress and maternal shock. Can be a life-threatening emergency

- Risk for women who labour with a scarred uterus is 2.1 per 1000. Risk is further increased by use of oxytocin and more so with prostaglandins

RECOGNITION AND ASSESSMENT

- If any of the following occur in a woman with a scarred uterus, call middle grate obstetrician (ST3–7 or equivalent e.g. staff grade, clinical fellow) or consultant obstetrician to review woman urgently

Symptoms and signs of scar rupture

- Abnormal electronic fetal monitoring (EFM) trace

- Acute onset of scar tenderness

- Severe abdominal pain especially if between contractions

- Breakthrough pain during epidural analgesia

- Chest or shoulder tip pain or sudden onset of shortness of breath

- Vaginal bleeding or haematuria

- Maternal tachycardia, hypertension or shock

- Undue maternal distress, agitation

- Cessation of previously efficient uterine activity

- Loss of station of presenting part

IMMEDIATE MANAGEMENT

Scar rupture suspected

General

- Ensure maternal resuscitation is managed effectively

- Stop oxytocin if in progress

- Administer oxygen at maximum flow

- Crossmatch four units of blood urgently

- Insert a second large-bore, cannula

- Assist mother into left lateral position with tilt

- Inform consultant obstetrician

- Call anaesthetist and theatre team urgently

- Anticipate a sick baby and call neonatal crash team, which must include a senior clinician

Specific treatment

- If woman fully dilated, perform vaginal instrumental delivery immediately

- If not favourable for instrumental delivery, obtain informed consent for laparotomy and possible hysterectomy and perform a grade 1 emergency caesarean section – see **Caesarean section** guideline

- See **Postpartum haemorrhage** guideline

Issue 3
Issued: April 2015
Expires: April 2017

SUBSEQUENT MANAGEMENT

Scar rupture confirmed (not simple dehiscence)

- Call consultant obstetrician and consultant anaesthetist

- It may be possible to repair uterus. Hysterectomy or subtotal hysterectomy may be required

- Method of repair depends on nature of tear, degree of haemorrhage and woman's future fertility wishes

- Give broad spectrum IV antibiotics – according to local Trust policy

- Provide mother with high dependency care – see **High dependency care** guideline

Communication

- Explain events fully to woman and family including implications for future pregnancies

- Report clinical incident using local incident reporting system

Issue 3
Issued: April 2015
Expires: April 2017

ANTENATAL CARE

- Women who have history of an uncomplicated lower-segment transverse caesarean section and an otherwise uncomplicated pregnancy with no contraindications to vaginal birth, discuss options of VBAC or elective caesarean section

- Discuss previous birth experiences with woman. Take her wishes into account and document discussion in maternal healthcare record

- Review notes or request information from other hospital (if applicable) to obtain details of previous caesarean section

- To enable woman to make informed choice, give VBAC leaflet (if available locally) during antenatal period, which includes risks of repeat caesarean section and risks of scar rupture in labour

- Obstetrician will agree mode of delivery with woman before expected/planned delivery date (ideally by 36 weeks' gestation) and document individual management plan for labour

- if labour occurs before planned caesarean section, record woman's choice

> *Rates of hysterectomy and blood transfusion increase in women who have had ≥2 previous caesarean births*

Contraindications to VBAC

- Previous upper segment caesarean section – advise woman to give birth by elective caesarean section

- previous uterine incision other than an uncomplicated low transverse caesarean section incision

- Previous uterine rupture

- >2 previous caesarean deliveries

- Women with this history who wish to consider vaginal birth should be assessed by a consultant obstetrician with full access to details of previous surgery (if possible)

- When considering planned VBAC in woman with a twin gestation, adopt a cautious approach

INTRAPARTUM MANAGEMENT

- If local practice, establish IV access

- FBC and group and save

- A midwife competent in the care of high-risk conditions should care for woman during labour on a one-to-one basis, and inform delivery suite co-ordinator of any change in care

- Inform middle grade obstetrician (ST3–7 or equivalent e.g. staff grade, clinical fellow) that woman is on labour ward

- When woman in labour, give oral ranitidine 150 mg approximately 6–8-hrly

- If mode of delivery not previously agreed, consultant obstetrician to discuss with woman

INDUCTION OF LABOUR

- Consultant obstetrician will discuss risks with woman

- two-to-three–fold increased risk of uterine rupture and around 1.5-fold increased risk of caesarean section in oxytocin-induced and/or augmented labours compared with spontaneous labour

- higher risk of uterine rupture where prostaglandins used for induction of labour

- no increased risk of uterine rupture with induction using transcervical balloon catheter – see **Transcervical catheter induction** guideline

- Women who wish to have VBAC should be seen by consultant in antenatal clinic at 40 weeks and offered membrane sweep, discussion on mode of delivery and place of labour and an individualised and documented plan of delivery

- Vaginal examination can help to assess the favourability for induction and method of induction

- membrane sweeping is not contraindicated

Monitoring

- Once labour established, record careful serial assessments on partogram – see **Labour management** guideline

- Continuous electronic fetal monitoring (EFM) to detect signs of impending rupture, following the onset of contractions (see **Electronic fetal monitoring** guideline)

- In uterine rupture, an abnormal EFM trace is present in 55–87% of cases

Augmentation

- Although not contraindicated, decision to prescribe oxytocin must be made by consultant obstetrician after obstetric assessment and discussion with woman

- If prescribed, titrate oxytocin to the ideal contraction frequency rate of 3–4 in 10 min

> *If no progress in labour in the presence of adequate uterine activity and oxytocin augmentation, proceed to caesarean section as soon as possible*

Uterine rupture

- See **Uterine rupture** guideline

- Observe for symptoms and signs including:

- tenderness, or sudden pain over scar within abdomen, sudden cessation of uterine activity (especially if pain breaks through epidural) or shoulder tip pain

- bleeding vaginally not associated to cervical dilatation

- easily palpable fetal parts

- haemodynamic instability (low BP, raised pulse, feeling unwell, unresponsive)

- EFM changes showing sudden bradycardia or changes to variability

- loss of station of the presenting part

- If any of the above detected, inform middle grade obstetrician (ST3–7 or equivalent e.g. staff grade, clinical fellow) and delivery suite co-ordinator immediately

INTRODUCTION

- The incidence of breech presentation decreases from approximately 20% at 28 weeks' gestation to 3–4% at term when most babies will turn spontaneously to the cephalic presentation

After discussion with woman, consultant obstetrician will advise on mode of delivery. Document discussion and decision clearly in maternal healthcare record

DEFINITION

- Presentation of fetal buttocks or feet in labour

ANTENATAL MANAGEMENT

- Unless contraindicated, offer external cephalic version (ECV) preferably at 36–38 weeks' gestation

- Advise women with unfavourable clinical indicators of the increased risks to them and their babies if considering vaginal breech delivery

CONTRAINDICATIONS TO ECV

Absolute

- Lower segment caesarean section (LSCS) to be performed for another reason (e.g. placenta praevia)

- ≥2 previous LSCS

- Severe oligohydramnios (ECV usually impossible)

- Multiple pregnancy

- Fetal compromise

Relative

- Intrauterine growth restriction (IUGR)

- Uterine scar

- Known Rh isoimmunisation

- Antepartum haemorrhage

- Women in labour

INDICATIONS FOR VAGINAL BREECH DELIVERY

- Maternal choice (in some units, vaginal breech delivery is offered as an option)

- Extreme prematurity

- Stillbirth

- Second twin

- Rapid progressive labour with insufficient time to perform caesarean section

Favourable features

- Estimated fetal weight between 2–3.8 kg

- Clinically adequate pelvis (presenting part engaged)

- Complete breech presentation

INTRAPARTUM MANAGEMENT

- Perform planned vaginal breech deliveries on consultant-led delivery unit with access to facilities for emergency caesarean section

- Planned vaginal breech delivery must only be undertaken by an experienced obstetrician or experienced midwife

- In an emergency situation, midwife is expected to manage delivery

First stage of labour

- On admission, inform middle grade obstetrician (ST3–7 or equivalent e.g. staff grade, clinical fellow), who will discuss with consultant obstetrician

- Full intrapartum assessment by midwife/middle grade obstetrician

- Abdominal palpation

- Commence continuous electronic fetal heart monitoring. If difficulty recording fetal heart rate abdominally, use fetal scalp electrode applied to buttock only

- Vaginal examination

- Insert cannula and obtain blood for full blood count (FBC) and group and save

Issue 3
Issued: April 2015
Expires: April 2017

- Offer woman choice of analgesia for labour and delivery

- for planned vaginal breech delivery, consider epidural analgesia

- Artificial rupture of membranes (ARM) not usually performed due to risk of umbilical cord prolapse

- Avoid oxytocic drugs

- Avoid use of fetal blood sampling during labour on a breech presentation

> **If delay or fetal compromise at any stage during labour, consider caesarean section**

- Passage of meconium cannot be relied upon as an indicator of fetal distress

Second stage of labour

- Inform middle grade obstetrician (ST3–7 or equivalent e.g. staff grade, clinical fellow)/consultant and ask to attend for second stage of labour

- Until presenting part is below the level of the ischial spines, discourage bearing down

- Undertake urinary catheterisation

- Perform vaginal examination to confirm fully dilated cervix (particularly important preterm) and position of breech

- In active second stage, assist into lithotomy position to enable breech delivery

- Call anaesthetist and theatre team

- Request attendance of a neonatologist. See **Cardiopulmonary resuscitation of the newborn** guideline

Delivery

- Allow natural descent of fetal buttocks – **hands off**

- Evaluate the need for episiotomy; consider waiting until fetal anus visible over fourchette

- Ensure fetal spine rotates uppermost during delivery

- Encourage mother to actively push, to aid baby's natural descent and 'minimise handling'. Do not pull on baby's body or legs, flexed breech legs usually deliver spontaneously

- If assistance required to deliver legs, once popliteal fossa visible, release legs by flexing at the knees

- Observe for anterior scapula and allow time for arms to release spontaneously. If assistance required, hook arms down from the elbow. If this is not sufficient, two fingers can be passed over the shoulder to push the humerus across the chest

- if other shoulder does not deliver spontaneously, repeat manoeuvre

- Allow baby to hang until nuchal line visible. Deliver head using Mauriceau-Smellie-Veit manoeuvre – a combination of maxillary and occiput pressure

- If an obstetrician is conducting delivery they may decide to deliver the head using forceps

- Perform active management of the third stage

Post delivery

- Obtain cord blood for venous/arterial testing and record result – see **Umbilical cord sampling** guideline

- Debrief parents

- Arrange neonatal review for newborn and infant physical examination (NIPE)

Delayed engagement of the after coming head in the pelvis

- Second attendant will perform supra pubic pressure to assist flexion of the head

Obstructive delivery of the after coming head

- If conservative methods fail, consider tocolysis, McRoberts manoeuvre, symphysiotomy or caesarean section

Preterm breech

- Discuss mode of delivery of a preterm breech on an individual basis with woman and partner wherever possible

- If labour well established, there may be no choice but to proceed to a vaginal delivery. In this case, **most senior person available** must carry out the delivery. Otherwise, where possible, an ultrasound scan assessment of the fetal size will be performed and a decision on the mode of delivery made by on-call consultant obstetrician

- Where there is entrapment of after coming head, consider lateral incision of cervix

Documentation

- Ensure clear documentation of:
- procedure
- help summoned
- names and grades of personnel attending
- timing of events
- communication with woman
- Follow local incident reporting procedure

Issue 3
Issued: April 2015
Expires: April 2017

RECOGNITION AND ASSESSMENT

- Diagnosis of DVT and pulmonary embolism in pregnancy can be challenging because of the physiological changes that occur. Many of the classical symptoms of venous thromboembolism can occur in a low risk pregnancy

Symptoms and signs

- Leg pain
- Swelling
- Oedema
- Tenderness
- Change in leg colour
- Increased skin temperature
- Low-grade pyrexia
- Raised WCC

Investigations

> *If DVT suspected, start treatment with low molecular weight heparin (LMWH) until diagnosis*

- Compression or duplex ultrasound is the first line diagnostic test for DVT in pregnancy. It is non-invasive, highly sensitive (97%) and specific (96%) for symptomatic proximal vein DVT, but is less accurate for isolated calf DVT
- if ultrasound negative and there is a low level of clinical suspicion, discontinue anticoagulant treatment
- if symptoms suggestive of PE, see **VTE – Pulmonary embolism** guideline
- If iliac vein thrombosis suspected (back pain and swelling of entire limb), consider magnetic resonance venography

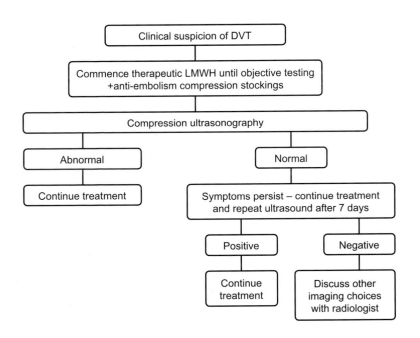

Clinical suspicion of DVT
↓
Commence therapeutic LMWH until objective testing +anti-embolism compression stockings
↓
Compression ultrasonography
↓
- **Abnormal** → Continue treatment
- **Normal** → Symptoms persist – continue treatment and repeat ultrasound after 7 days
  - **Positive** → Continue treatment
  - **Negative** → Discuss other imaging choices with radiologist

TREATMENT

General

- Adequate analgesia
- Compression stockings
- in initial management of DVT, elevate leg and fit graduated elastic compression stocking to reduce oedema

Specific

- Blood for FBC, INR, APTT
- If platelet count <75 x 10^9/L, seek advice from on-call haematologist before starting anticoagulation
- If platelet count ≥75 x 10^9/L, prescribe subcutaneous LMWH (Dalteparin or Enoxaparin – according to local practice)

Initial anticoagulant treatment in pregnancy

- In clinically suspected DVT, administer LMWH (Dalteparin or Enoxaparin – according to local practice) at doses below until objective testing excludes diagnosis
- In women with renal impairment, seek advice on dosage from haematologist

Therapeutic dose of LMWH

Initial dose	Early pregnancy weight (kg)				
	<50	50–69	70–89	90–110	>110
Dalteparin	5000 units 12-hrly	6000 units 12-hrly	8000 units 12-hrly	10,000 units 12-hrly	Calculate dose on individual weight 1 mg/kg 12-hrly
Enoxaparin	40 mg 12-hrly	60 mg 12-hrly	80 mg 12-hrly	1000 mg 12-hrly	

Monitoring LMWH treatment

- If woman has not been given unfractionated heparin, monitoring for heparin-induced thrombocytopenia is not required
- If early pregnancy weight <50 kg or >90 kg and woman has bleeding problems, renal impairment, or massive PE, discuss need for anti-Xa monitoring with consultant haematologist

Maintenance treatment

- Choose one of the following two options after discussion with consultant haematologist
- therapeutic LMWH for 8–12 weeks followed by prophylactic dose for the rest of the pregnancy and at least 6 weeks postnatally **OR**
- therapeutic LMWH throughout pregnancy and at least 6 weeks postnatally

Anticoagulant therapy during labour and delivery

- Discontinue LMWH maintenance therapy 24 hr before planned delivery
- Advise woman that once she is established in labour or thinks she is in labour, no further heparin or other anticoagulant should be injected
- Do not administer regional anaesthetic or analgesic until at least 24 hr after last dose of therapeutic LMWH

Issue 3
Issued: April 2015
Expires: April 2017

Administration of LMWH and use of epidural/spinal anaesthesia

- Before carrying out regional anaesthetic procedures, (i.e. insertion of epidural catheter or administration of a spinal injection) you must record when the most recent dose of LMWH was given and follow the steps below:

- wait 12 hr after a prophylactic dose of LMWH

- wait 24 hr after a therapeutic dose of LMWH

- After insertion/removal of an epidural catheter (or after insertion of a spinal anaesthetic) you must review the time that has elapsed before administering a dose of LMWH. LMWH can be given postnatally while epidural is *in situ*:

- a thromboprophylactic dose of LMWH can be given 4 hr after removal of epidural catheter

- Do not remove epidural catheter within 10–12 hr of most recent LMWH

Postnatal anticoagulation

- Continue therapeutic anticoagulant therapy for at least 6 weeks postnatally and until at least 3 months of treatment has been given in total. Offer a choice of LMWH or oral anticoagulant (warfarin)

- If starting warfarin, provide woman with counselling and an oral anticoagulant booklet. Document in book with follow-up appointment on discharge

- Heparin and warfarin are not contraindicated in breastfeeding

- If woman chooses to commence warfarin postpartum, avoid until at least the third postnatal day

- Daily INR testing is recommended during the transfer from LMWH to warfarin to avoid over-anticoagulation

DISCHARGE AND FOLLOW-UP

- Offer women who have been diagnosed with VTE during pregnancy or postnatal period a 6 week–3 month postnatal appointment with consultant haematologist

RECOGNITION AND ASSESSMENT

- Diagnosis of DVT and pulmonary embolism in pregnancy can be challenging because of the physiological changes that occur. Many of the classical symptoms of venous thromboembolism can occur in a low risk pregnancy without VTE

Symptoms and signs

- Dyspnoea
- Collapse
- Chest pain
- Haemoptysis
- Faintness
- Tachycardia
- Tachypnoea
- Raised JVP
- Reduced PaO_2 +/- $PaCO_2$
- A high clinical suspicion is critical to diagnosis

> *If PE suspected, start treatment with low molecular weight heparin (LMWH) until diagnosis*

Investigations

- Oxygen saturation
- ABG
- ECG
- Chest X-ray (with fetal shielding)
- if another cause for pleuritic chest pain found, treat appropriately
- Discuss choice of ventilation perfusion (VQ) lung scan or computerised tomographic pulmonary angiography (CTPA) with radiologist
- advise woman that small risk to fetus associated with low-dose perfusion scan or CTPA (1:280,000) compared with a very high risk of maternal death (1 in 7) associated with untreated PE during pregnancy

- A diagnosis of DVT may indirectly confirm a diagnosis of PE and, since anticoagulant therapy is the same for both conditions, further investigation may not be necessary. This would limit the radiation doses given to woman and fetus and is the approach for all suspected non-massive PE (normal chest X-ray, ECG and haemodynamically stable)
- Continue anticoagulant treatment until PE definitely excluded

TREATMENT

Massive life-threatening PE in pregnancy

- Resuscitate and give oxygen
- Involve multidisciplinary resuscitation team including consultant physician, consultant obstetrician, consultant anaesthetist and radiologist
- If PE confirmed, urgent CTPA or portable ECHO and team decide whether IV unfractionated heparin, thrombolytic therapy or thoracotomy and surgical embolectomy appropriate
- IV unfractionated heparin is preferred in massive PE because of its rapid effect and extensive experience of use – 75 units/kg bolus (based on booking weight) followed by 18 units/kg/hr to maintain APTT of 2–3 times average laboratory control value
- in women with renal impairment, seek advice on dose reduction from haematologist

General

- Resuscitate and give oxygen to maintain SpO_2 between 94–98%
- Adequate analgesia

Issue 3
Issued: April 2015
Expires: April 2017

Specific

- Blood for FBC, INR, APTT
- If platelet count <75 x 10⁹/L, seek advice from on-call haematologist before starting anticoagulation
- If platelet count ≥75 x 10⁹/L, prescribe subcutaneous LMWH (Dalteparin or Enoxaparin – according to local practice)

Initial anticoagulant treatment in pregnancy

- In clinically suspected DVT or PE, administer LMWH (Dalteparin or Enoxaparin – according to local practice) at doses below until objective testing excludes diagnosis

Therapeutic dose of LMWH

Initial dose	Early pregnancy weight (kg)				
	<50	**50–69**	**70–89**	**90–110**	**>110**
Dalteparin	5000 units 12-hrly	6000 units 12-hrly	8000 units 12-hrly	10,000 units 12-hrly	Calculate dose on individual weight
Enoxaparin	40 mg 12-hrly	60 mg 12-hrly	80 mg 12-hrly	1000 mg 12-hrly	1 mg/kg 12-hrly

Monitoring LMWH treatment

- If woman has not been given unfractionated heparin, monitoring for heparin-induced thrombocytopenia is not required
- If early pregnancy weight <50 kg or >90 kg and woman has bleeding problems, renal impairment, or massive PE, discuss need for anti-Xa monitoring with consultant haematologist

Maintenance treatment

- Choose one of the following two options after discussion with consultant haematologist
- therapeutic LMWH for 8–12 weeks followed by prophylactic dose for the rest of the pregnancy and for at least 6 weeks postnatally

OR

- therapeutic LMWH throughout pregnancy and for at least 6 weeks postnatally and until 3 months treatment has been given in total

Anticoagulant therapy during labour and delivery

- Discontinue LMWH maintenance therapy 24 hr before planned delivery
- Advise woman that once she is established in labour or thinks she is in labour, no further heparin or other anticoagulant should be injected
- Do not administer regional anaesthetic or analgesic until at least 24 hr after last dose of therapeutic LMWH

Administration of LMWH and use of epidural/spinal anaesthesia

- Before carrying out regional anaesthetic procedures, (i.e. insertion of epidural catheter or administration of a spinal injection) you must record when the most recent dose of LMWH was given and follow the steps below:
- wait 12 hr after a prophylactic dose of LMWH
- wait 24 hr after a therapeutic dose of LMWH

- After insertion/removal of an epidural catheter (or after insertion of a spinal anaesthetic) you must review the time that has elapsed before administering a dose of LMWH. LMWH can be given postnatally while epidural is in situ:

- a thromboprophylactic dose of LMWH can be given 4 hr after removal of epidural catheter

- Do not remove epidural catheter within 12 hr of most recent LMWH

Postnatal anticoagulation

- If no bleed, re-start anticoagulation treatment 4 hr after delivery

- Continue therapeutic anticoagulant therapy for at least 6 weeks postnatally and until at least 3 months of treatment has been given in total. Offer a choice of LMWH or oral anticoagulant (warfarin)

- If starting warfarin, provide woman with counselling and an oral anticoagulant booklet. Document in book with follow-up appointment on discharge

- Heparin and warfarin are not contraindicated in breastfeeding

- If woman chooses to commence warfarin postpartum, avoid until at least the third postnatal day

- Daily INR testing is recommended during the transfer from LMWH to warfarin to avoid over anticoagulation

DISCHARGE AND FOLLOW-UP

- As part of medical discharge, offer women who have been diagnosed with VTE during pregnancy or postnatal period a 6 week–3 month postnatal appointment with consultant haematologist

Issue 3
Issued: April 2015
Expires: April 2017

INTRODUCTION

- Venous thromboembolism (VTE) is up to ten times more common in pregnant women than in non-pregnant women of the same age and can occur at any stage of pregnancy but the puerperium is the time of highest risk

RISK FACTORS

Pre-existing

- Previous VTE
- Thrombophilia (see **Table** below)
- Age >35 yr
- Obesity (BMI >30 kg/m2) pre- or early pregnancy
- Parity >3
- Smoking
- Medical co-morbidities e.g. sickle cell disease, cardiac disease, proteinuria >3 g/day, inflammatory bowel disease, joint disease or myeloproliferative disorders
- IV drug user
- Gross varicose veins
- Paraplegia

New onset/transient

- Hyperemesis/dehydration
- Ovarian hyper-stimulation syndrome
- Admission, immobility (>4 days bed rest) e.g. symphysis pubis dysfunction restricting mobility
- Surgical procedure in pregnancy or puerperium
- Albumin below normal range for pregnancy

Ongoing individual risk assessment

- Infection (requiring antibiotics or hospital admission) e.g. pneumonia, pyelonephritis
- Long-haul travel (>4 hr)

Heritable	Acquired
- Antithrombin deficiency	- Lupus anticoagulant
- Protein C deficiency	- Anticardiolipin antibodies
- Protein S deficiency	
- Factor V Leiden	
- Prothrombin gene variant	

Obstetric

- Multiple pregnancy
- Assisted reproductive therapy
- Pre-eclampsia
- Prolonged labour >24 hr
- Mid-cavity or rotational operative vaginal delivery
- Caesarean section
- Excessive blood loss (>1 L) or requiring transfusion

VTE RISK ASSESSMENT

- Complete local risk assessment proforma for thromboprophylaxis at: -
  - antenatal booking
  - antenatal admission
  - risk assessment in labour
  - post-delivery

Perform VTE risk assessment and initiate appropriate action using local VTE assessment tool

Special circumstances requiring thromboprophylaxis

- Unless contraindicated, the following require thromboprophylaxis:
- massive PPH
- severe PET
- severe post dural puncture headache

MANAGEMENT

General

- Do not allow woman to become dehydrated
- Encourage to mobilise
- if immobilised, arrange leg exercises as soon as possible after surgery
- Consider using regional anaesthesia if appropriate (risk of VTE is higher with general anaesthesia)
- Risk assessment (using local VTE assessment tool) to ascertain if further measures necessary [e.g. graduated compression stockings, low molecular weight heparin (LMWH)]
- In some circumstances, mechanical compression devices will be used e.g. where graduated compression stockings or LMWH contraindicated

Graduated compression stockings (GCS)

- On admission, offer GCS, unless contraindicated (see below)
- Staff trained in the use of compression stockings should show woman how to wear them correctly and monitor their use
- Encourage women to wear GCS from admission until they return to their usual levels of mobility

Contraindications to GCS

- Peripheral vascular disease
- Severe dermatitis
- Recent skin graft
- Leg deformity
- Peripheral neuropathy

Low molecular weight heparin (LMWH)

- If risk of bleeding, give thromboprophylaxis in 2 divided doses
- One week thromboprophylaxis for most women but 6 weeks if high risk, including previous VTE

High thromboprophylaxis dose

- If high thromboprophylaxis dose required, seek advice from haematologist
- Any woman weighing >90 kg (booking weight) receiving high dose low molecular weight thromboprophylaxis – check anti-Xa levels
- anti-Xa cannot be carried out as an urgent test and result may not be available for 2–3 days but would at least guide subsequent treatment
- If woman at very high risk of VTE or previously on long-term anticoagulation – Refer to thrombosis clinic or seek advice from haematologist

Standard thromboprophylaxis dose

Early pregnancy weight	Dalteparin	Enoxaparin
<50 kg	2500 units once daily	20 mg daily
50–90 kg	5000 units once daily	40 mg daily
91–130 kg	7500 units once daily	60 mg daily
131–170 kg	10000 units once daily	80 mg daily
>170 kg	75 units/kg/day	0.6 mg/kg/day

Issue 3
Issued: April 2015
Expires: April 2017

Contraindications to LMWH

- Active bleeding
- Platelet count <75 x 10^9/L
- Coagulopathies
- Renal impairment
- Uncontrolled hypertension (>200 systolic or >120 diastolic)
- Allergy to heparin/LMWH

Administration of LMWH and use of epidural/spinal anaesthesia – Precautions

- If vaginal bleeding or labour begins, stop LMWH
- Discontinue prophylactic LMWH on day of planned delivery
- High prophylactic dose or therapeutic dose – change to prophylactic dose on day before planned delivery
- Before carrying out regional anaesthetic procedures, (i.e. insertion of epidural catheter or administration of a spinal injection) you must record when the most recent dose of LMWH was given and follow the steps below:
- wait 12 hr after a prophylactic dose of LMWH
- wait 24 hr after a therapeutic dose of LMWH
- After insertion/removal of an epidural catheter (or after insertion of a spinal anaesthetic) you must review the time that has elapsed before administering a dose of LMWH. LMWH can be given postnatally while epidural is *in situ*
- a prophylactic dose of LMWH can be given 4 hr after removal of epidural catheter
- Do not remove epidural catheter within 12 hr of most recent LMWH
- If regional technique was traumatic or had a bloody tap, consider skipping the next dose of LMWH

INDICATIONS

- Any pregnant woman at term who is suitable for low-risk care in labour

- Women who request waterbirth against advice must be seen by consultant obstetrician and supervisor of midwives as soon as possible

Preparation and cleaning of pool

- Follow local infection control measures

FIRST STAGE LABOUR

Before entering pool

- Labour should be established

During labour

> **Do not leave woman unaccompanied in the pool**

- Fill pool to level of mother's breasts

- In warm, humid environment, encourage fluids to prevent maternal dehydration

- Monitor maternal temperature closely and discontinue use of pool if a rise of 1°C above baseline

- Monitor and record fetal heart rate with watertight sonic aid

- Monitor water hourly to maintain a temperature that is comfortable for the woman but do not exceed 37.5°C at **any time**

- Keep water clear of debris

- Use only nitrous oxide and oxygen (50/50) for analgesia in waterbirth

SECOND STAGE LABOUR

- Two midwives must be present at birth

- Delivery is mainly a 'hands off' procedure and control of the head is therefore unnecessary as immersion in water appears to facilitate slow crowning

- Following delivery of the head, the trunk should be expelled with the next contraction. If this does not happen, encourage mother to stand up and deliver baby in air

- Deliver baby completely under the water and bring to the surface immediately with the face uppermost

> **If baby delivered in air, do not allow to re-enter water**

THIRD STAGE MANAGEMENT

- Placental delivery and control of bleeding will be dependant on maternal consent for active or physiological management

- Observe for deviations from the norm

- Manage signs of maternal compromise as per local practice

Postpartum haemorrhage

- Maternal compromise may indicate postpartum haemorrhage

- Estimation of blood loss is difficult in water and therefore it is estimated at < or >500 mL

- For major obstetric haemorrhage – see **Antepartum haemorrhage** guideline and **Postpartum haemorrhage** guideline

- If perineal suturing required, allow one hour for oedema to reduce

- Suturing should be completed within 2 hr

REASONS FOR MOTHER LEAVING POOL

- Fetal distress

- Meconium stained liquor

- Failure to progress

- Mother becomes unsuitable for low-risk care e.g. pyrexia, bleeding, fainting

- Maternal request or to pass urine

- Maternal request for analgesia other than inhaled (50/50) nitrous oxide and oxygen

- Excessive water contamination

Issue 3
Issued: April 2015
Expires: April 2017

EVACUATION POLICY

- In the event of an emergency where mother unable to make an assisted rapid exit from birthing pool
- Call for help, using emergency call bell system
- Rapidly fill pool to allow woman to float to the top. Support her head above water
- Use evacuation equipment available locally (kept in birthing pool room at all times)
- Ensure a minimum of four adults (ideally six) two or three each side of the pool
- Remove foot of bed and bring bed to foot of birthing pool
- Evacuate mother from pool with two consecutive manoeuvres, first to bottom edge of bed, a short pause and then complete manoeuvre onto bed
- **Remember** – the woman will be wet and at risk of hypothermia – dry immediately

Issue 3
Issued: April 2015
Expires: April 2017

Issue 3
Issued: April 2015
Expires: April 2017

Issue 3
Issued: April 2015
Expires: April 2017